Access Your Online Support Material

Supporting Autistic Children with SLCN in the Early Years is accompanied by a number of printable online materials, designed to ensure this resource best supports your professional needs

Go to https://resourcecentre.routledge.com/books/9781041043072 and answer the question prompt using your copy of the book to gain access to the online content.

SUPPORTING AUTISTIC CHILDREN WITH SLCN IN THE EARLY YEARS

This fully revised second edition is an essential resource for anyone supporting young Autistic children with speech, language and communication needs (SLCN). Packed with practical, evidence-informed advice and guidance, it adopts a neuroaffirmative approach that shifts the focus away from changing the child and towards understanding and adapting the environment.

Drawing on Autistic-led research and contemporary theories and concepts, including Gestalt Language Processing, monotropism, the Double Empathy problem, alexithymia and interoception, the book translates key concepts into practical strategies that can be embedded within everyday routines, interactions and educational settings. Helping readers develop a deeper understanding of how and why Autistic children communicate, interact and experience the world around them, the book offers:

- An introduction to Autism and SLCN, breaking down key research into easily digestible chunks
- Detailed case studies and examples throughout
- Practical activities and resources, including planning sheets and activity suggestions
- Easy-to-follow chapters focusing on the classroom environment, communication, social interaction, play and behaviour.

Full of evidence-based practical strategies, this manual is essential reading for staff supporting Autistic children with SLCN in an early years setting. It is also valuable reading for other allied health professionals and parents.

Jennifer Warwick is a speech and language therapist passionate about working with Autistic children and young people. She works as part of a multi-disciplinary team assessing and providing intervention for children, young people and their families. Jennifer is a joint author of the *Early Sociocognitive Battery* published by Hogrefe. She is an advisor to the Royal College of Speech and Language Therapists (RCSLT) for Autism and social communication and is a Research Champion for RCSLT. Jennifer volunteers for the Le Jeune Charity for Children with Down Syndrome and is a part time clinical tutor at Anna Freud, part of University College London.

nasen

Helping Everyone Achieve

nasen is a professional membership association that supports all those who work with or care for children and young people with special and additional educational needs. Members include SENCOs, school leaders, governors/trustees, teachers, teaching assistants, support workers, other educationalists, students and families.

nasen supports its members through policy documents, peer-reviewed academic journals, its membership magazine *nasen Connect*, publications, professional development courses, regional networks and newsletters. Its website contains more current information such as responses to government consultations.

nasen's published documents are held in very high regard both in the UK and internationally.

For a full list of titles see: https://www.routledge.com/nasen-spotlight/book-series/FULNASEN

Other titles published in association with the National Association for Special Educational Needs (nasen):

Supporting Children with Complex Needs: An Evidence-Informed and Holistic Approach to Create Connectivity in the Classroom
Julia Lindley-Baker and Laura Mills
2026/pb: 978-1-032-29314-1

Unlocking Playtime Potential: Reducing Conflict and Maximising the Positives of Unstructured Time in Schools
Amelia Roberts
2026/pb: 978-1-003-40889-5

The SEN Practitioner: Status, Skills and Support
Tristan Middleton
2026/pb: 978-1-003-62384-7

Supporting Autistic Children with SLCN in the Early Years: A Practical Resource for Professionals, 2ed
Jennifer Warwick
2027/pb: 978-1-041-04307-2

SUPPORTING AUTISTIC CHILDREN WITH SLCN IN THE EARLY YEARS

A PRACTICAL RESOURCE FOR PROFESSIONALS

Second Edition

Jennifer Warwick

Routledge
Taylor & Francis Group
LONDON AND NEW YORK

Designed cover image: © Getty Images

Second edition published 2027
by Routledge
4 Park Square, Milton Park, Abingdon, Oxon, OX14 4RN

and by Routledge
605 Third Avenue, New York, NY 10158

Routledge is an imprint of the Taylor & Francis Group, an informa business

First edition published by Routledge 2020

British Library Cataloguing-in-Publication Data
A catalogue record for this book is available from the British Library

ISBN: 9781041043171 (hbk)
ISBN: 9781041043072 (pbk)
ISBN: 9781003627760 (ebk)

DOI: 10.4324/9781003627760

Typeset in Open Sans
by Newgen Publishing UK

Access the Support Material: https://resourcecentre.routledge.com/books/9781041043072

CONTENTS

ACKNOWLEDGEMENTS

With huge thanks to Mia Marks, Nari Ertem, Maeve Hoxha and Dr Stephanie Ewan for their contributions to this manual. They are invaluable and will help so many others.

Thank you also to my colleagues Rachael McCarthy and Annmarie Sims for your contributions and for working so collaboratively and generously.

Thank you also to Kieran Rose (the Autistic Advocate) for giving permission to share a key image included in this manual.

Thank you always to Isla, Ruby and Alex.

Finally a huge thanks to all the children, young people and families I have learnt so much from along the way.

1

Understanding Autism: theories and shifting perspectives

Chapter 1 provides the following:

- An introduction to this manual and how to use it
- Consideration of the neurodiversity paradigm and why this is important
- An overview of Autism to support your understanding
- Relevant theories and key concepts
- Case study examples

Introduction

This manual has been written for people working with Autistic children in the early years environment. The manual will also be useful for parents and carers of an Autistic child and anyone wanting to learn more about Autism in children under five. You may be a teaching assistant, teacher, SENCO, health-care professional or student. Regardless of your background I hope you find a wealth of information and practical ideas to challenge your thinking and foster curiosity. One of the key aims of this second edition is also to help break down harmful stereotypes and I hope that the discussion and examples may shift your thinking about Autism and empower you to approach situations and the children and families you meet with joyful curiosity.

Whilst I have tried to avoid technical terms and heavy theoretical descriptions, it is important to have a good grounding of Autism and current thinking around Autistic thinking styles. It is also important to continue to stay curious and seek out new perspectives as they arise.

DOI: 10.4324/9781003627760-1

Thinking around Autism continues to be a changing landscape as new research and perspectives arise. As professionals working with Autistic children and their families, we have a responsibility to be curious, to act without judgement and to take on new ideas. Whilst I urge you to read the theories and take time to digest them, continue to look towards those with lived experience to gain deeper understanding of what it is really like to be Autistic. In my years working as a speech and language therapist (SLT) I have learned more about Autism from Autistic people than anywhere else.

Since the publication of the first edition one key observation relating to my own practice is that we can cause more harm than good by having too many unachievable goals, too many prescriptive targets in a learning plan of what a child will or won't do. Positive change comes from a place of shared understanding and collaboration, from being partners in change and most importantly from observing and listening without jumping to conclusions and judgements. The parents' perspectives included in the next chapter highlight the importance and need for professionals to really listen to the views and experiences of parents and to work in partnership with them.

In my 20 years as an SLT I have seen that SLTs are great 'fixers' often coming in with many strategies and ideas. Whilst all of these are well meaning they might not be the right approach. As educators and professionals working with Autistic children and their families, we can do a disservice by not taking the time to build relationships, to collaborate and really understand before jumping to strategies. I have always advocated the approach of 'change the environment not the child' and in my practice I generally see this as by far the most effective way of working with Autistic children and young people. This perspective very much fits with Dr. Luke Beardon's (2017) Autism + Environment = Outcome framework which we talk about in more detail later in this chapter.

When using this manual, I would set you a challenge to think about how you can be an 'ally' to Autistic people in the work you do. In the last edition I talked about the importance of 'spreading awareness', ten years on we need to do more and do it differently. If you are reading this, I imagine that you have a genuine curiosity and desire to help. One of the biggest shifts in my practice since really listening to Autistic voices and learning (and continuing to learn) about the neurodiversity paradigm is the shift from wanting to 'change' and just 'build skills' to being an ally and championing the voices of the Autistic people I work with. I would encourage you to read the parent perspectives in the next chapter and use the themes raised in them as tools to start discussions with your colleagues. If you are looking to learn more about Autism from the perspective of Autistic people, there are so many brilliant Autistic authors out there! From my own perspective I would recommend Pete Wharmby, Kieran Rose and Emily Katy, but there are many, many more. I have included several of their books and resources in the references section of this chapter.

There is a lot of information in this manual! I would encourage you to read the current chapter thoroughly to digest the key theories and concepts. They may seem heavy but understanding these is crucial in enabling non-Autistic people to better understand the experience of Autistic people. Chapters 2–6 have a practical focus that you can re-visit according to what the children you work with need at specific times. The manual is designed to be re-visited and used in as practical a way as possible.

Each chapter has a range of activity sheets to accompany it. These are practical ideas with strategies of how to support a child. It is important to note that they do not replace advice from an SLT or other professional but can provide ideas for activities and support. They are written in a simple and user-friendly way and are designed to be accessible. They can be copied and included in a child's planning and learning journey to make sure that they are accessible.

Activity sheets can be used for a whole nursery approach or to use one on one with an individual child. The activities can also be used in groups.

What is in your toolbox?

In my work, the analogy of a toolbox is something I come back to time and time again. It is a framework that I have found very helpful in supervision and in discussions with parents, educators and other professionals as well as in my own practice. Considering 'what tools I need in my toolbox' at any particular time is a helpful starting point to equip me to best support the children and families I work with. I would encourage you to think of your individual toolbox and what you need in it to help support and understand the children you work with. The toolbox analogy is helpful as it acknowledges we will need different tools at different times and these tools will change over time. I also think about the parents and children I work with and what tools they may need at any particular time.

Activity

Think about your toolbox. What do you need more of? What do you need less of? Draw it out and add ideas as you go through the chapter!

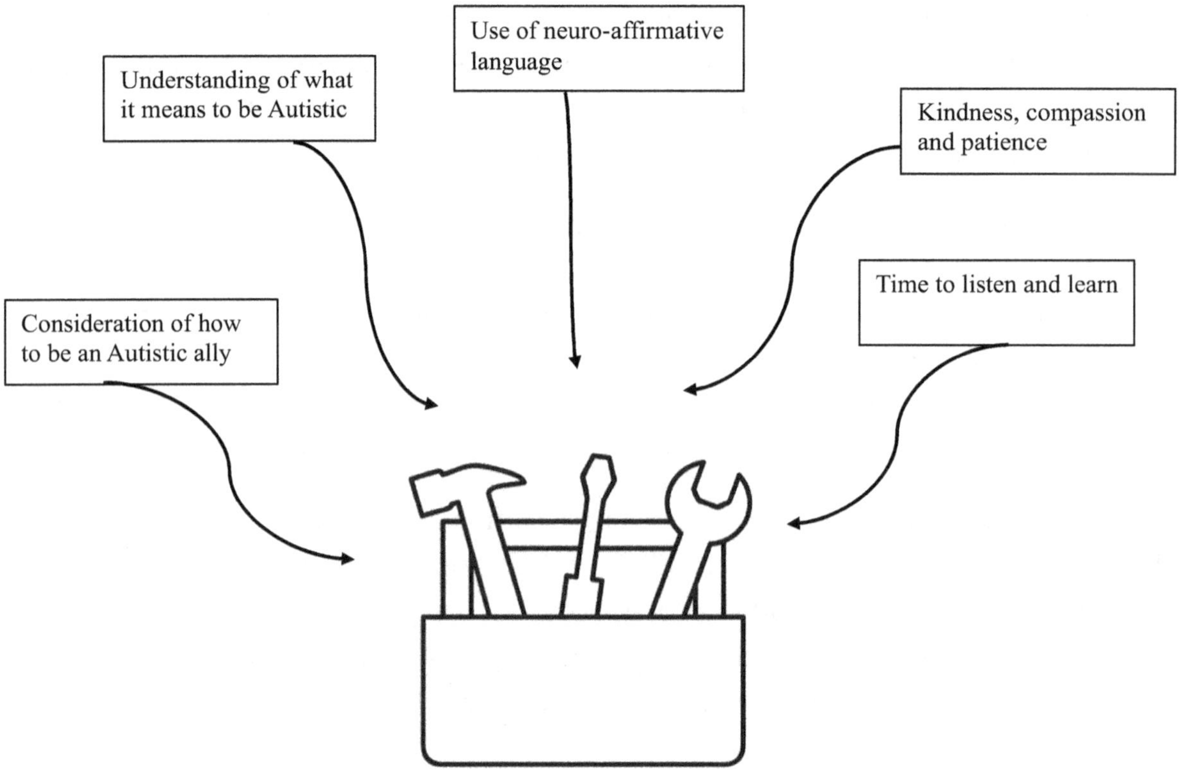

Figure 1.1

Let's look at Figure 1.1, which shows a visual example of a toolbox.
Since the original writing of the first edition in 2018 there have been shifts in how we think and talk about Autism and neurodivergence generally. Shifting perspectives have been a driving factor in the need to update and rethink parts of this manual in order for it to remain current and make sure it stays relevant for years to come.

Some of these shifts are really significant and obvious, including changes in terminology and language as well as the identification of new and better theories of how we conceptualise Autism. Other shifts may seem more subtle including shifts in language and the move away from 'pathologising' to 'understanding', of talking about differences rather than difficulties.

Shifts in thinking are important and represent a need to do better for Autistic people. As a clinician my work has always sought to empower the children, families and professionals I work with. I trained as an SLT in 2003 when the narrative around 'disability' was very much shifting from a medical model to a social model, but at this time assessment and intervention for Autistic children often sought to 'change' and 'normalise' patterns of communication, play and behaviour. Approaches to support communication often came from a 'neurotypical' perspective of what communication is so clinicians under the guise of being helpful sought to 'increase eye contact' or 'develop pretend play'. Whilst the last edition sought to take into account the views and thoughts of Autistic people and parents of Autistic children at the time of writing, a lot of thinking (whilst well intended) was still very much rooted in a deficits based perspective.

Over the last ten years, my practice has been shaped hugely by the influence of Autistic people, by the neurodiversity paradigm and through adopting a genuine curiosity and culture in my practice for continual learning. My biggest source of learning in the last ten years has been the Autistic teenagers I have the privilege to work with and meet through the diagnostic process who are able to so clearly describe what the world is like for them. This has been very impactful in my journey as a clinician. Listening to Autistic voices is powerful and I would encourage you to seek these out.

I have no doubt that in ten years' time there will be further shifts in our thinking as a society and I certainly hope that our understanding of neurodivergence as a whole is further on than where it is now. It is helpful to first turn to the neurodiversity paradigm to understand more about the context of shifting perspectives.

Neurodiversity paradigm

The neurodiversity paradigm is the idea that there are many natural ways for human brains to develop and work, none are better than the other, but some brains are more common. The neurodiversity paradigm recognises the inherent strengths that different brains and thinking styles bring. Differences such as Autism, Attention Deficit Hyperactivity Disorder (ADHD), dyslexia and other neurodevelopmental conditions are seen as normal variations of the human mind, not deficits or illnesses that need to be fixed. When we think of different brains in this way, we can see that challenges often arise not because a person is broken, but because the world is designed with only one type of brain in mind. When the environment, other people's expectations and the support doesn't fit with a person's way of thinking and being, difficulties can increase. The neurodiversity paradigm is a useful and important framework as it recognises both strengths and challenges while respecting neurological differences as part of who a person is. It emphasises support and understanding over fixing, it values lived experiences and focuses on improving quality of life not changing someone. Importantly, it does not deny that neurodivergent people can experience real distress and disability. A key message to take away from the neurodiversity paradigm is that of differences rather than deficits and the idea that better outcomes for neurodivergent people firmly come from acceptance plus support, rather than more pressure to conform.

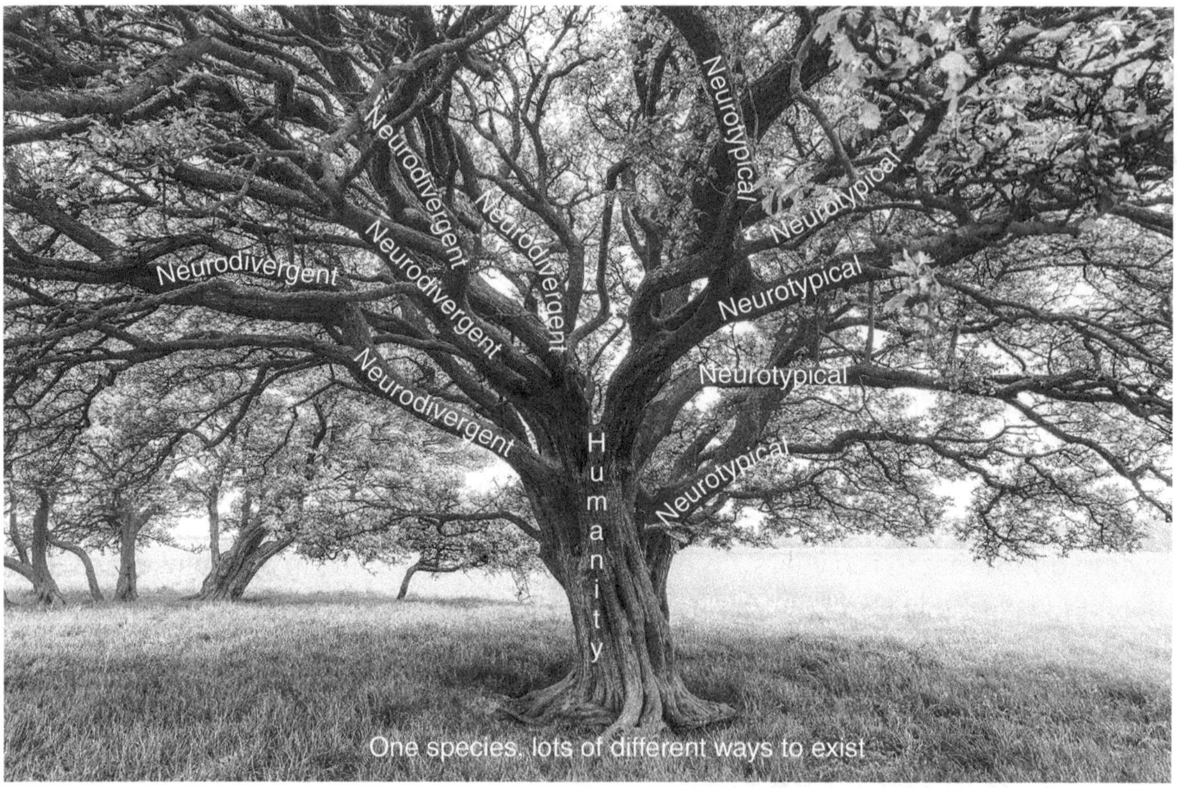

Figure 1.2 One species, lots of different ways to exist. Image by wirestock on Freepik.

In Figure 1.2, with kind permission from 'the Autistic Advocate', Kieran Rose highlights the intrinsic value of all brains. We are one species with many different ways to exist. Many people (including me) use the analogy of neurodiversity being a bit like biodiversity. I use this when I am talking to children about their brains. Wouldn't it be boring if we just had one type of plant or animal? We need rich and varied plant and animal life to make it a good planet. In the same way we also need lots of different types of brains.

What is Autism?

Our understanding of Autism is changing all the time. We can define Autism as a neurodevelopmental condition that impacts how people experience the world. There are two core areas associated with Autism and to get a diagnosis there needs to be differences in both of these areas (see Table 1.1):

- Communication and social interaction
- Restricted and repetitive interests and behaviours (RRBIs)

When we are thinking about what Autism is, it can also be helpful to think about what Autism isn't; Autism is not a learning difficulty although it can be accompanied by learning differences in some children. Autism is not a mental health condition although Autistic people may experience higher levels of anxiety and have poor mental health. Autism is not caused by parenting but sadly I continue to work with lots of families who are made to feel like it is. Current evidence supports the view that Autism is genetic. This is, however, very complicated and there is no one gene that causes Autism. Autism is not caused by taking paracetamol in pregnancy or vaccines. Myths around causes of Autism can create huge damage and it is important to be informed but recognise understanding is changing all the time. We do know that Autistic children grow up to be Autistic adults and that Autism is life long, it is not a condition that can be 'cured' or grown out of. Through understanding and embracing neurodiversity we can do a lot in celebrating all ways of seeing the world.

The idea of a 'spectrum' can be problematic as it can imply a line which someone has a static point on. It can imply that someone may be more or less Autistic; in fact one of the most common questions I am asked at the point of diagnosis is 'where do you think my child is on the spectrum?', 'are they at the mild end or severe end?'. The idea of a 'point on a line' also fails to take into account the impact of the environment. For any child, particularly of nursery age, the environment can have a huge impact on how they are in any situation. When we give an Autism diagnosis often people ask, 'what level of Autism are they?'. Whilst the current diagnostic criteria do include three levels of support (Level 1, Level 2 and Level 3), my experience in the UK is that these are not often used and whilst the intention may be around giving support to children, grouping children into broad categories is not always helpful and doesn't tell us much about their individual needs.

In my experience rather than thinking of a diagnosis as a fixed point on a line or a certain level, it is more helpful to think of a young person's individual profile of Autistic characteristics and strengths and differences. Some people find the analogy of a pie chart helpful in conceptualising Autism, the idea being that each section of the pie represents different areas associated with Autism. Each child will have a unique pie and the segments in it will shift over time. Another analogy that we use in our parent group is that of a constellation with each point representing different areas associated with Autism (sensory, communication, interests). The points on the constellation can be joined together with a line to create a unique shape representing the child's profile of strength and areas of difference that again will change over time.

When we think about Autism it is important to also consider co-occurring conditions and think about the impact of these on a child. Autism can often co-occur with other neurodevelopmental conditions such as Attention Deficit Hyperactivity Disorder (ADHD), dyspraxia, language disorder, as well as areas of difference with sleep, toileting, eating and learning. A comprehensive assessment in line with NICE (2017) guidelines (typically led by a neurodevelopmental paediatrician) is an important starting point as considering the wider context is crucial, particularly in young children who may not be able to comprehensively describe what is going on for them and understand holistically the bigger picture. As Autism advocate Dr. Stephen Shore (2004) has famously stated, 'If you've met one person with autism, you've met one person with autism', highlighting the considerable variability that exists within the autistic population. This quote remains relevant, particularly when we think about Autistic children and young people. I often meet families and educators who hold a particular view of an Autistic child which is different from their own child or the child they are currently working with. Fixed views about Autism can block curiosity about a child, therefore having a clear yet flexible viewpoint can be a helpful starting point. Whilst understanding of neurodivergence and Autism has shifted in society there continue to be a lot of negative and unhelpful stereotypes, often these are used in a very general way, for example 'he's definitely not Autistic he's got great eye contact!' or 'she doesn't have any problems with routines or fussy eating' so she's definitely not Autistic. The parent perspectives in Chapter 2 highlight how these stereotypes still can have a harmful impact and their impact can be long lasting.

A lot of people I come into contact with when I run training or parent workshops tell me that it can be confusing as the Autistic population, like any population, can vary hugely. Whilst this can feel complex and overwhelming the first thing to recognise and acknowledge is that every Autistic child will be different and that is ok! Our job is to be curious in getting to know them and think flexibly in our approach. We need to come from a place of genuine curiosity rather than a narrower perspective where we may jump to the wrong conclusion.

Activity

Challenge yourself to think of any stereotypes that you hold around Autism. Why do you think it is important to challenge these stereotypes?

Words matter

The words we use to describe Autism and Autistic children matter. Words can have a long-lasting impact both from a positive and negative perspective. It is therefore important that we pay attention to them and choose them with care. In my own work I continue to develop this and recognise that this process is ongoing and would encourage you to do the same. I recently met a friend of a parent of nursery age who talked about a conversation with their child's nursery where staff had talked endlessly of their child's 'struggles' without a single mention of a strength, imagine being that parent!

In reading this book you will see language that seeks to affirm and describe rather than to stigmatise and pathologise. Subtle shifts in language can have a real impact, remember we are talking about people's children.

When we think about language another really key point is to consider how children hear us talking about them. Lots of parents I work with will highlight how stressful it is getting to the nursery pick up to be given a comment of *'Mum he's had a bad day...'*. Making time to talk about a child not within their ear shot, even if they look like they are not listening, is really important.

Activity

Challenge yourself to think about how you and colleagues describe the children you work with. Try to make small shifts one word at a time. We want to replace words like problem, dysfunction, atypical difficulty and symptoms with more helpful terms. For example, think about describing a child's differences rather than difficulties.

Tip

Make sure that you use a communication book that goes between home and nursery so that you can write down important observations and information to share with parents. Remember to include strengths and positives. This means key information can be shared without a child having to listen at the end of the day when they just need to leave the setting.

Table 1.1 Strengths and differences frequently seen in Autistic children

Communication and social interaction
Differences in verbal communication can include: - A delay in language acquisition but equally some children can have language that appears advanced for their age with a strong vocabulary particularly in relation to interests. - A different pattern of language development, more echolalia and learnt language - see more in Chapter 4 on Gestalt Language Processing. - Differences in use and understanding of tone, volume, rhythm and rate of speech, including speaking in accents. - Talking a lot but finding back and forth conversations harder. - A literal understanding and use of language which can make it hard to understand when people around them are not clear and direct. - Difficulties with abstract and ambiguous language and instructions. - Interaction that can appear different. Autistic children may show differences with their play, they may prefer to play in parallel, show a deep focus on favoured activities and show distress when play is interrupted. - Strengths in an honest and direct communication style. - Generally a stronger visual than auditory processing; visual processing is an area of real strength. Differences in non-verbal communication can include: - Using or understanding gestures differently. - Different eye contact and facial expressions. It is important to acknowledge that there is no 'right or wrong way' to show expressions and all forms of communication are valid.
Restricted and repetitive behaviours and interests
Autistic people may show: - A strong memory and eye for details. - Strengths in visual processing. - Special interests that may seem very in depth. This may be knowing everything about a particular TV programme or a specific topic, e.g. knowing lots of in-depth facts about the solar system. - Strong and special interests - being able to focus on these is important and comforting. - Preference for routines and predictability - this can mean that it is harder for Autistic children to manage change. - Repetitive movements including flapping hands and rocking. In some children these can be very subtle. - Enjoyment in playing with the same activities again and again. Sensory differences come under the umbrella of RRBIs: - These include being over or under sensitive to sensory information in the environment. This may be sounds, smells, touch or visual and may be a comfort for a young person. For Autistic children there may be distress caused by certain stimuli, e.g. an unpredictable bell ringing at school or the hand dryer going off unexpectedly. - Joy in sensory experiences and preference for play that aligns with sensory preferences.

Strengths and differences - what we see

Table 1.1. above considers the differences we see associated with the core characteristics of Autism. This list is not exhaustive but provides a starting point of characteristics that you may notice in the Autistic children you meet and work with. Just remember that each child will have different combinations of core characteristics, and these can look different in different environments. Try to keep an open mind and don't get stuck on stereotypes. These characteristics vary widely between children and may present differently depending on the environment.

Activity

Think of children that you work with, note down areas of strength and areas of difference that you have noticed. Keep these in mind when we turn now to look at relevant theories and key concepts.

Getting a diagnosis

The process of getting an Autism diagnosis can be long and stressful for many parents. The parent perspectives later in the next chapter outline how not everyone has a smooth route to get to this point. Some parents have a clear early understanding that their child may be showing some developmental differences and are keen to proceed and access support whereas others may not feel that a diagnosis is the right thing for their child at this time. It is important to be familiar with how diagnostic services work in your area, any referrals that you may need to complete and any useful services available locally including parent groups that offer support. It is important also to acknowledge that even if parents may seem ready for the diagnosis, it can still be an extremely emotive and stressful process and it is important that you are equipped to support them in this journey.

Tip

Think of how you would feel if it was your child. When you are talking to parents or identifying areas of difference remember to describe strengths as well as needs. If you have noticed areas of difference that could be related to Autism in your setting, remember the following:

- Talk to parents and ask them what happens at home. Often children can present differently in different situations, and this information can be helpful to know.
- Start with the positives: 'What's going well?'
- Record observations and planning; this documentation can be helpful when applying for support later on if it is required.
- Remember to leave the diagnosis to the child development team. I've heard 'he's definitely got Autism' many times. Whilst a child may have many features and may get a diagnosis, it's not helpful to label without a diagnosis. It is not always helpful for parents to hear this.

- See the child and understand the whole picture rather than getting overly focussed on a label.
- If a parent asks you questions that you don't know the answer to, don't feel tempted to say something misleading like, 'Don't worry ... he will be fine', instead acknowledge how you can seek support together and make a plan.
- Signpost parents to local speech and language therapy services and local support available. Encourage parents to go to their general practitioner and discuss their concerns.
- Unfortunately, there is a lot of misleading information out there about Autism which can lead to parents going away feeling confused and upset. Making sure you know reputable sources to signpost parents to is important.
- If your area has a local child development service, find out what the process is in terms of making a referral and who can do this. If you are able to provide this information to parents in a timely way, this can be supportive.

A paediatrician, SLT or clinical psychologist is usually involved in the assessment. The assessment will likely involve direct observation and assessment with the child, a structured parental history and gathering of information from a different context such as a nursery.

For more information about Autism generally and the process of Autism assessment, you can signpost families to the National Autistic Society (www.autism.org.uk).

Relevant theories and key concepts

When I run training and parent groups, we spend time talking about relevant theories and perspectives. Often participants feedback that this is one of the most helpful components in enabling them to understand their children and the children they work with. The next section turns to consider relevant theories and concepts to help us make sense of Autism. It does not include every theory in existence to explain Autism, but key theories and concepts are provided to give a grounding in Autistic thinking styles.

Double Empathy Theory

The Double Empathy Theory comes from Dr. Damian Milton (2012) and is a helpful way to think about Autism in line with the neurodiversity paradigm. Historically there was an idea that Autistic people struggled with understanding other people and empathy, however lots of Autistic people and researchers noticed that this really wasn't the case, and that Autistic people generally understand other Autistic people well. I very much see this reflected in my work in the friendships and connections that young Autistic people have. The theory challenges the historical view and says communication problems between Autistic and non-Autistic people go both ways, not just one way. So, in essence, blaming an Autistic person for not understanding a non-Autistic person is wrong. It's a bit like different cultures understanding each other where there are different signals, customs and systems.

Double Empathy Theory says:

- Autistic people understand other Autistic people well.
- Non-Autistic people understand other non-Autistic people well.
- Problems can happen when Autistic and non-Autistic people try to understand each other.
- It's not that one group doesn't have empathy, it's because each group has a different way of thinking, communicating and seeing the world.
- The 'double' part comes from the idea that both sides may not feel understood – confusion and frustration can go both ways and both sides may struggle to read each other, resulting in communication breakdown. A good example of this is that an Autistic person may value and favour a direct clear communication style whereas a non-Autistic person may see this as rude and prefer a more subtle communication style with more implied meanings and hints. Both styles of communication are valid and reasonable; neither side is wrong

Double Empathy Theory is really important because it sees a shift from perspectives that blame or overly pathologise Autistic people. It comes from a place of mutual understanding, adjustment and support and emphasises that society should make changes and adapt and not expect Autistic people just to fit in.

When I think about Double Empathy Theory and how it impacts my practice the image that often comes to mind is a bridge. I think to myself, how can we 'bridge the gap'? Holding this in mind with the children you work with is really important and helps us to consider helpful adjustments and support rather than an expectation that a child will fit in. When we make adjustments and use strategies that support mutual understanding, we tend to see much better outcomes all round. A common example I see is children struggling with the transition to starting a new class or setting. When we hold Double Empathy in mind, we may make adjustments such as preparing a child with a photo social story, a visit before starting to have a look around, a staggered starting time, a box of favourite toys, a clear timetable showing when home time is, thorough discussion with parents around strengths and differences and individual preferences. When we expect a child to just 'fit in' there tends to be none of this, and an expectation that they will just 'get used to the routine' which can often result in tearful partings from parents. Often staff will kindly let a parent know that a child is 'fine when you are gone', however it may be the case that a child is so shut down and focussed on a predictable activity they look fine but are not.

Monotropism

When I first heard about monotropism (Murray et al., 2005, 2021), I had a real 'ah ha' moment; I often find the same happens when I talk about the theory to parents or teachers. The theory of monotropism really helps us to understand why a child behaves in a certain way and why certain things are easier and some are harder. Monotropism is a theory that Autistic people came up with to explain how many Autistic people focus their attention and energy very deeply on a small number of things. A polytropic brain (which neurotypical children typically have) can spread attention across lots of things; this contrasts with a monotropic brain which tends to focus intently for longer periods and lock into several interests. Monotropic brains are a bit like a torchlight (focussing intently on a small area) whereas a polytropic brain is more like a lamp (lighting up lots of things all the same). Both thinking styles are valid, neither is better or worse than the other; they are just different. Having a monotropic brain can bring huge strengths but it can make some things harder, especially in a school environment where the curriculum (even in early years) is built for being able to easily shift attention and focus on lots of things a little bit rather than one or two intently.

Monotropism can mean that a child may:

- Get very deeply absorbed in particular interests, toys or topics that they love
- Do really well with tasks that need focus, detail and persistence
- Find it difficult when there are interruptions to what they are doing
- Need to finish an activity and move onto something else (particularly if this is less motivating)
- Need time to help them finish and switch between things

Lots of older students I work with are able to show incredible focus on topics that motivate them but find it really hard to engage with smaller tasks that don't hold interest or motivation, often those around them can find this confusing or frustrating. The theory of monotropism can really help to explain Autistic experiences to non-Autistic people including special interests and why these are so important, needing a routine and feeling overwhelmed by too many demands at once. In an early years setting it can help us shift our narrative about a child from 'he won't do it' to 'his attention is on something else'. For young Autistic children with a monotropic attention style it is hard being in an environment where you are expected to switch your attention between lots of different topics rather than just focussing on the ones you are interested in. When we understand monotropism it becomes clear how important it is to include an Autistic child's interests in learning and activities within the early years setting. This is essential in supporting engagement.

Activity

Think about your environment and how many times a child is expected to shift their attention during the day. What and why do you think this is hard for the children you work with?

Weak Central Coherence

Uta Frith described the Weak Central Coherence Theory of Autism in 1989. Whilst this theory is quite old and the word 'weak' seems a little misplaced, it still remains relevant in explaining some elements of Autistic thinking. In its simplest sense Central Coherence is a term that means being able to see 'the bigger picture', as in the ability to draw meaning from lots of details. Autistic children and young people that I meet often show huge strengths in their ability to notice the small details. Kids I work with are often detail driven which means that they may notice small details that non-Autistic people miss, they may have very strong abilities in recognising patterns, they may have a very strong memory for details and also a deep focus on detail and wanting to know all the details about something that is motivating to them. This thinking style brings many strengths, however it can mean that Autistic children find it easier to 'zoom in' to the small details but can find it harder to 'zoom out to see the bigger picture'. It is important to remember that Weak Central Coherence describes a way of thinking and is not a deficit. This perspective fits with the principle that Autistic thinking is 'different but not broken' and acknowledges diversity in thinking. It can make sense of a child's focus on particular details and interests so is therefore helpful to be aware of.

Alexithymia and interoception

Understanding Alexithymia and interoception is another useful way that we can help non-Autistic people make sense of the Autistic experience. A child who experiences Alexithymia may feel emotions strongly but have trouble noticing, naming or explaining them. It's not that the child doesn't have feelings, it's that their feelings can be hard to recognise or put into words. You may see a child who finds it hard to say how they feel even if they have good language skills, a child who may use physical descriptions instead of emotion words. You might also see big emotion reactions that can seem to come 'out of nowhere' as well as children who experience difficulties with understanding the emotions of others; this can sometimes lead to reactions that look like they 'don't quite fit' with the situation. A little boy I worked with used to laugh when other children cried, staff tried to talk to him in terms of his behaviour not being kind. This approach didn't work as it failed to take into account that he didn't really understand the situation and how to respond.

Interoception is the ability to notice what's happening inside your body – in simple terms interoception helps a child to understand their body's messages. As adults we know that a tightening chest may mean anxiety, or a rumbling tummy means hunger. For young Autistic children it can be difficult to always sense hunger, thirst, needing the toilet, pain, tiredness or emotions. Interoception can be harder for some Autistic kids, so they might not realise or be able to put these body sensations into words. This can impact them in their daily life in many different ways.

Communicating how you feel is complicated for many children but for some Autistic children, emotions can feel like confusing body signals instead of clear feelings. For example, they might notice a sore tummy, tight chest or feeling 'too full', but not realise this means they are anxious, sad or frustrated. Often teenagers I work with describe how emotions all blur together and that the physical sensations they experience are all the same. Older teens have described how separating out feeling anxious and feeling excited can be difficult and it being tricky to pinpoint what a particular sensation means. Understandably this can lead to feeling very overwhelmed. Deciphering these feelings is complex and even harder when you are younger. Knowing about Alexithymia and interoception is helpful for educators and professionals because it means that we can understand more about emotion regulation and how to support this.

Supporting emotion regulation is an important part of early intervention but all too often in my experience there is an emphasis on the child needing to communicate how they feel rather than a motivation to look to the environment and understand more what may be causing difficulties with emotion regulation. Approaches where a child needs to point to a picture of how they feel or communicate this doesn't take into account the impact of Alexithymia and interoception. Regulation happens within the moment and in the environment. More on this later!

Masking

Masking occurs when Autistic people try to hide or change their natural behaviours to fit in with others. I have encountered stereotypes that only older Autistic children and teenagers mask and it is not something we see in younger children, which is absolutely not the case. In the parent perspectives in Chapter 2, Mia describes her daughter as a 'master of disguise' and highlights how staff working with her were not aware of the difficulties she was experiencing because of the level of masking. Masking in young children can appear in many ways. It might look like copying how other children play or talk, forcing eye contact, holding back stimming (like hand-flapping) or staying very quiet to avoid attention. Masking often happens because the child wants to be accepted or avoid getting in trouble and it can happen without a child even realising. I've met older teens who have only realised that masking is not something everyone does when they have completed a masking questionnaire as part of the assessment. When I talk to Autistic children and young people about their masking we often use the analogy of the swan. The swan glides along on the surface and its difficulties are not seen, but underneath the water line the swan is paddling hard. This unseen paddling is exhausting and can take its toll on a child. We know that masking is exhausting and can have a significant impact on children, young people and their families.

As well as masking we often see children who are 'holding it together', this is also known as restraint collapse. This can be illustrated by the fizzy cola bottle analogy where the bottle is shaken all day with the lid kept tightly on (this is the restraint bit). Only when the child gets home and the lid comes off the bottle there is usually a big explosion (the release of stress and the collapse). This occurs when a child is under stress but containing it until they get home. Generally a child 'holding it together' is using all their energy to manage noise, change and the many demands in the day. They may appear calm and compliant at nursery but when they are home (where they feel safe) and the stress is relieved there may be huge meltdowns and shutdowns. Parents may see a very different picture than what is reported in the educational setting. All too often I hear parents being dismissed or blamed when this occurs or the behaviour outside of education being seen as a separate problem or something the child has learnt or can control. In some cases where there has been a real lack of listening and collaboration, families have been made to feel that this is 'their issue' because there are 'no difficulties here' in the setting. I have been to settings to observe children where there are no concerns from staff but lots of distress and dysregulation after school. I have noticed that children of this age may be very vigilant watching and scanning the behaviours of others, they may be following the rules but not actively engaging. Other subtle signs may also include increased fatigue and sensitivity as the day progresses.

Tip

Really listen to parents when they are describing very different behaviours at home than what you see in the education setting. Be curious to hear the experiences rather than dismissing them.

Preference for sameness and predictability

In a deeply confusing and sometimes overwhelming world predictability and consistency can really help Autistic children to feel safe and secure. In my work with parents and educators I often find myself asking the question 'how can we make this more predictable?' When things happen in a predictable and familiar way Autistic children tend to feel safer and more comfortable. Knowing what is coming next helps an Autistic person's brain to feel organised and calm. Routines, predictability, familiarity and consistency help Autistic children manage uncertainty. This is one of the reasons that strategies like visual timetables, social stories and scripts can be really helpful in building understanding of new situations and what is happening as part of new routines.

Older young people I work with describe how difficult it is when plans are changed, or they aren't informed of something happening out of their routine like a dental appointment or Mum's friend coming over after school. To non-Autistic people it can seem like a lot of information but having the information in advance is really important to ensure the world feels more secure and safe. Before I meet children and young people (and Autistic adults) for the first time I will send a picture or a video with some information about what we will do to reduce uncertainty. This always helps to reduce anxiety by making the situations seem a bit more predictable.

I often hear that children need to 'manage change better' or 'become more flexible' or 'just get used to it'; these perspectives can be very harmful and fail to understand how important and powerful predictability is in supporting Autistic children. I would argue that first and foremost we need to be making the environment as predictable and consistent as possible to ensure that Autistic children feel secure and safe. This might mean the same morning routine or having the same activity every day after lunch. It also means thinking carefully about what is coming up so as to give clear warnings and information when something different will be happening.

We all engage in familiar activities as a way to recharge and reduce stress, often this might be coming home from work, having the same drink and watching a familiar TV programme. It's easy to see how comforting this could be. For an Autistic child this is really no different. I would ask: does a strong preference for the same toy or food or leisure activity really matter, especially if it is not having any negative impact on a child?

In the children you work with you might see:

- A child wanting things done in the same way each time
- Upset when plans change, especially if this is unexpected
- Strong attachment and connection to routines or objects
- A child that needs extra time or support to help them adjust to changes

The importance of special interests

We know that special interests are very important for Autistic people. With that torch-like monotropic focus it is easy to see how Autistic brains are drawn into topics of interest.

In trainings and conferences I have attended, I have often heard the quote 'I have never met an Autistic person who was depressed when engaged in their special interest'. Whilst it is not clear who originally said this, the sentiment really resonates and highlights the importance of special interests to Autistic children and young people. Later in this book when we talk in more detail about communication and social interaction we always come back to including special interests and the power of this in building a connection. Tuning into a child's special interests and preferences is always a good starting point.

Justice sensitivity

Justice sensitivity or a strong sense of right and wrong is often seen in Autistic young people. I have no doubt that many of the Autistic teens I have met will go on to do incredible work as a result of the fact that they are driven by a real sense of justice. Whilst this is an admirable quality it can make it very difficult to make sense of the behaviour of others, especially when they do not behave in the way that is expected. For younger children justice sensitivity can show up as a heightened awareness of the rules and fairness. This is often accompanied by a big reaction when something happens that is perceived as unfair or breaking the rules. It is important to be aware of this so that children are not viewed as 'overreacting' or having out of proportion reactions.

Sensory preferences

Everyone is talking about sensory! We often hear the phrase that Autistic children 'are very sensory' or 'sensory seeking'. However, in reality we are all sensory beings, and we all experience sensory preferences or likes and dislikes in our daily lives. An example my occupational therapist (OT) colleague always uses is that of two children on the trampoline, one has a recent diagnosis of Autism and the other is neurotypical. Both children are jumping happily on the trampoline. For the neurotypical child they 'just like jumping', for the Autistic child they are 'sensory seeking'. Whilst both observations may be valid, we need to be careful not to over pathologise and to view sensory experiences in isolation. We also need to view sensory experiences in the context of the environment. Take the example of a fire alarm. If we know that a fire alarm goes off every Thursday at 11:00am and we are used to it and hear it every week we have a minimal response to it. If a fire alarm goes off at random when we are in a stressful situation like waiting for a job interview we are much more likely to startle and have an amplified reaction. We know that Autistic people experience the sensory world differently, which means that everyday sensory information may be amplified or reduced. This means that lights, sounds, smells, touch and taste may seem a lot, very overwhelming or harder to register. In my daily life there are many sensory experiences that I don't like: I don't like the noise of nails on a blackboard, I don't like the smell of bubble gum and the sight of yoghurt has always made me feel sick. However, I don't have to encounter these on a regular basis, so my sensory dislikes don't really impact me in my day-to-day life in a significant way. If you are an Autistic child and the smell of lunch or the sound of the tidy up song are unbearable this can be problematic as you will hear these every day throughout the day.

Understanding how the sensory world impacts a child is an important step to understanding and supporting them. My OT colleague describes this as 'putting on our sensory goggles' to try and decipher what is going on for a child in any particular environment. We need to understand what experiences a child likes and which ones are problematic for them so we can provide support and accommodations, and most importantly so we can adapt the environment. Understanding an individual child's sensory likes and dislikes can also be very powerful in supporting their ability to engage in play and communicate; essentially, we communicate and engage in things we like so this is important.

It is important not to view 'sensory' as separate to the rest of the child. I met a child in a nursery recently where towards the end of the day he was getting tired and leaning on other children. The staff viewed this as a purely sensory behaviour and gave him a weighted cushion for his lap. We problem solved and came up with a strategy of modelling language around him being tired (remember a child may find this hard because of difficulties with Alexithymia and interoception) and offering a range of options including asking for a snack and having a rest. By problem solving we were able to understand what was going on for him and give him a wider range of tools to help in this situation.

Autism + Environment = Outcome

Dr. Luke Beardon's Autism + Environment = Outcome framework (2017) is a very powerful way to understand more about the Autistic experience. Sometimes known as 'the golden equation' it can help professionals, educators and parents understand that an Autistic child may thrive in some situations and environments but find others really difficult.

For early years educators and professionals working with Autistic children this is a powerful message and very much fits with the mantra 'Change the environment not the child'. The parent perspectives in Chapter 2 really fit with this. A key part of this framework emphasises that outcomes for Autistic children (and all Autistic people) are shaped by how well the environment that they are in understands, accommodates and responds to their Autistic way of being. Essentially the framework is saying:

- Autism is a difference not a problem
- The environment has a big impact on Autistic people and distress, difficulty or success result from interactions with the environment
- If we change the environment we change the outcome

Strengths

Autistic children have many strengths. I have had the pleasure of working with many wonderful Autistic children and young people and see the strengths an Autistic thinking style brings. This list is not exhaustive, but here are some that I have observed:

- A strong attention to detail in tasks and activities that are motivating
- Strong interests and passions
- Visual learning skills
- A strong sense of right and wrong
- A good sense of humour
- Motivation to learn about favoured topics

Using a child's strengths and interests is a great place to start in terms of understanding them and how best to support them.

Tip

I have been to many planning meetings involving education staff, parents and professionals that often become lengthy discussions about what a child is unable to do. Starting the meeting with strengths, what is going well, can totally change the tone of the meeting. Make sure that in any written learning plans or special educational needs and disability (SEND) support plans you start with areas of strength and then move onto needs.

Case study examples

Case studies are always a helpful way to consider the unique strengths and differences in Autistic children and to gain greater understanding of how even though children may share a common diagnosis their presentation and therefore the support and adjustments they need in the environment will be different. We turn now to look at the profiles and strengths of two different children who are both Autistic.

Name: Louie

Age: three years and six months

About Louie

- Louie is a joyful little boy diagnosed as Autistic when he was two and a half.
- Staff working with him feel that the diagnosis has helped them to understand him. They have been able to access relevant training and support. They have

had meetings to find out from parents what is working well at home and there is good communication between home and nursery through a communication book and monthly meeting of an hour.

- Louie knows lots of words, especially descriptive words. He communicates using short phrases, for example, 'red square'. Most of his phrases are to label things around him rather than to ask for things. Louie is a determined boy and often tries to get things himself, he is good at climbing and often does this very well to reach items that he wants. Sometimes when he can't communicate what he wants he can become frustrated. He will sometimes lead an adult's hand to items he wants.
- Louie repeats lots of words and phrases, he has a Gestalt Language Processing style of language development (more on this in Chapter 4).
- Louie follows the routine of the nursery; staff have noticed that he responds well to photos to support the routines. He can find it harder to manage when the routine changes. He doesn't always respond to spoken instructions.
- Louie absolutely loves playing with water and sand, he can do this for hours and he is very happy and calm pouring the water between a cup and a jug and letting the sand run through his fingers. He loves to watch this.
- Louie connects with adults and approaches them for hugs. He plays alongside his peers and sometimes he will lean on other children or gently push them and laugh.
- Louie does not like certain unexpected noises including the cries of other children, the hand dryer and adults singing. He will cover his ears and scream when these happen.

Strengths

- Louie learns new words quickly; he is musical.
- Louie has close family relationships and he is always very happy to be picked up. He loves tickling and chasing games with his parents.
- Louie is joyful and curious; he is interested in the world around him.
- Louie is able to focus on self-selected activities; his interests are highly motivating and comforting to him and are a powerful way to support him.

Name: Lucille

Age: four years and ten months

About Lucille

- Lucille is a bright and articulate young girl; she surprises those around her with her knowledge of animals and grown up words and phrases. She can talk a lot about topics that she is interested in and is very passionate about animals. Talking about these brings her a lot of joy.
- Her nursery did not have any concerns about her until her parents shared their issues regarding her behaviour at home. They were surprised that she had huge meltdowns every day when she got home.
- She recently received a diagnosis of Autism. At the time of diagnosis, the diagnostic team emphasised that Autistic girls may present differently from boys. They drew attention to the fact that Autistic girls may mask and internalise some of their difficulties, which can cause anxiety.
- Lucille is verbal and talks in long sentences. She loves animals and will talk at length about these; she finds it difficult to have conversations with other people that aren't about animals.
- Lucille sometimes uses language that she has learnt from a book or television programme. She uses phrases such as 'I do believe...' which gives her language a slightly formal quality. She knows a lot of facts about animals and she will often offer these as a way to start an interaction.
- Lucille can become distressed if she thinks that a rule has been broken; she often will try to reinforce what she believes are rules which other children can find difficult. For example, within the nursery environment children are allowed only two minutes on a bike, which is shown by a timer. If a child stays on slightly longer, Lucille becomes distressed and tries to pull him or her off.
- Lucille tends to seek out adults; she loves chatting to staff at nursery.
- Lucille watches the other children closely but sometimes seems unsure what to do.
- Lucille can cope with the day-to-day routine at home and nursery but can find it difficult to cope with changes to the routine. There is a school trip coming up, and staff are worried how Lucille will cope with this.

Strengths

- Lucille has a strong sense of right and wrong.
- She has wonderful language skills and an ability to absorb facts and information relating to her interests.
- She is interested in others and really enjoys chatting with adults.

Activity

Have you met children like Louie and Lucille? What do you notice in the children you work with? Jot down areas of strength and areas of need to build up a profile.

Chapter 1 summary

- Autism is a neurodevelopmental condition that impacts how a child sees the world. Each Autistic child that you meet will be unique but will have differences in the areas of social communication and interaction and RRBIs.
- Understanding how Autistic children see and experience the world is important for educators and professionals. We need to understand relevant theories and key perspectives to help us 'get in their shoes'.
- The neurodiversity paradigm and important theories like Double Empathy and monotropism help us to understand that Autism is a difference not a deficit.

References

Beardon, L. 2017. *Autism and Asperger Syndrome in Adults.* 2nd ed. Sheffield: Sheldon Press.

Frith, U. 1989. *Autism: Explaining the Enigma*. Oxford: Blackwell.

Milton, D.E.M. 2012. On the ontological status of autism: The 'double empathy problem'. *Disability & Society*, 27(6), pp.883–887.

Murray, D., Lesser, M. and Lawson, W. 2005. Attention, monotropism and the diagnostic criteria for autism. *Autism*, 9(2), pp.139–156.

Murray, D., Walker, N., Lawson, W., Hill, V., Pellicano, E. and Mandy, W. 2021. Monotropism: An interest-based account of autism. *Autism*, 25(6), pp.1501–1512.

National Institute for Health and Care Excellence (NICE). 2017. *Autism Spectrum Disorder in Under 19s: Recognition, Referral and Diagnosis* (CG128). Available at: www.nice.org.uk/guidance/cg128

Shore, S. 2004. *Ask and Tell: Self-Advocacy and Disclosure for People on the Autism Spectrum*. Olathe, KS: Autism Asperger Publishing Company.

Useful reading materials from Autistic authors:

Katy, E. 2025. *Girl Unmasked: How Uncovering My Autism Saved My Life*. London, England: Monoray (Octopus Publishing Group).

Kieran Rose also has many useful materials on his website: https://theautisticadvocate.com

Pearson, A. and Rose, K. 2023. *Autistic Masking: Understanding Identity Management and the Role of Stigma*. Brighton: Pavilion Publishing & Media Ltd.

Wharmby, P. 2023. *Untypical: How the World Isn't Built for Autistic People and What We Should All Do About It*. London: HarperCollins Publishers (Mudlark).

2

Understanding Autism: working together

Chapter 2 provides the following:

- In depth parent stories as an opportunity to reflect on the experiences of parents of young Autistic children
- Introduction to the iceberg model and how to use this as a tool to understand and problem solve what may be going on for a child in a particular moment

Parents' perspectives

Listening to parents is fundamental to ensuring strong relationships and a good foundation for collaborative support. I am endlessly grateful to the parents I have worked with over the years for helping me understand their children and what Autism means for them. I have asked parents that I work with to share their experiences with you. Their rich stories provide a really valuable insight and highlight strengths and differences as well as variability in provision and support.

Parent story 1

When they say a mother knows, she really knows. My son is now four and a half years old and I suspected he was Autistic from around the age of six months old. Close friends and family thought I was an anxious first-time mother or just bonkers! But I knew, and my son was officially diagnosed with Autism at two and a half years old.

Lots of people ask me how did you know? And it is a fair question particularly because my son is extremely well-behaved, always smiling, curious and overall a very happy and easy going child. My instinct was telling me that he was not sharing

DOI: 10.4324/9781003627760-2

his enjoyment with me in the way that I saw other children do with their parents. For example, he would look up at an aeroplane in the sky and stay fixed on it until it disappeared. I would see other children look at that same aeroplane and then look back at their parent as though they were telling their parent 'look Mummy/Daddy, I see an aeroplane'. As my son continued to develop, I also noticed that he was very much in his own world and would do things 'his way' in a repetitive manner. He could spin balls, roll cars forwards and backwards and line up toys perfectly for hours. He also went through a phase of being very restless in his pram and waking up and staying awake each night for 2–3 hours. Each phase was relatively short lived and while some of these traits are present in neurotypical children, my son was displaying more than one trait at the same time. What then cemented it for me was that his speech was delayed and he was also late to walk as he was bottom shuffling.

The first time my son was assessed by a neurodevelopmental paediatrician he was around 15 months and the doctor concluded that they were not concerned on the basis that he did all the activities really well. I definitely did not disagree that he performed really well but all I saw was a child who was looking down at the activity table throughout. He was then assessed again at age two where the neurodevelopmental paediatrician said Leo does have a number of Autistic traits but that he also has a number of strengths so they wanted to re-assess six months later which is when he was finally diagnosed.

What I have come to learn is that parents should always trust their instincts. What I battled with most is that it is not natural for a parent to focus on their child's challenges or difficulties. For me, my son was, and definitely still is, the most incredible person ever and I have always admired his dedication and perseverance to complete things in a certain way and how bright he is.

I can understand that some parents feel pressure to change the way their Autistic child may do things or how they behave towards certain people and this may be society putting a degree of pressure on us to do this. I used to feel slightly embarrassed if my son wouldn't say hello to someone or turn his back to them but it is truly ok and not everything links back to Autism, some children are just shy! This is an important balance when it comes to schooling. On the one hand it is helpful for the school to know about a diagnosis but on other hand, there is always a risk that a child's behaviours are attributed back to their Autism when in actual fact, it may just be typical four-year-old behaviour. We spent a lot of time researching schools and speaking to SENCOs (which I would recommend) and we feel very grateful that our school has been exceptionally supportive at getting to know our son and integrating him.

If possible, I would say that access to speech and language therapy (SLT) as early as possible can change a lot. SLTs are amazing not only at encouraging children to use their words to speak but also to improve the function of their language in social situations to help interact with peers and build friendships which can be a struggle for some children with Autism.

We also managed to procure an education, health and care plan (EHCP) for our son and I would recommend this for anyone who thinks that their child requires additional support in their education setting. However, it is important to remember that it is not about lowering barriers for children with Autism but rather removing obstacles which stand in the way of their hidden strengths.

Finally, there can be a lot of worry that comes with raising a child with Autism. In particular, one has to put their trust into an education setting and I have personally spent a lot of time wondering if he is ok. How will they encourage him to do something he doesn't want to do? Did he eat his food? What kind of future does he have? Will he work and be independent? And much more. As parents, we tend to always be 'one step ahead' of our children, which means that we are able to avoid situations which might be challenging for them and we protect them in this way. Ultimately I believe that Autism can be a wonderful thing because I see it in my own child but it needs support. Any support for a child with Autism should be designed to reduce or manage their anxiety levels. A more relaxed child will be more amenable to learning and interacting with peers. In the meantime, enjoy your child, keep up the fun and also celebrate their differences which can bring so much value to others.

Parent story 2: Mia Marks

I am the mother of Hazel, age seven, and Jack, age five. I know I am biased, but Hazel and Jack are such wonderful, brilliant children. Hazel is witty and has the most amazing attitude towards life. She is popular without wanting to be, wonderfully creative without trying to be, and the kindest, gentlest person I know. Every day, she wakes up ready for whatever the day will bring. Jack has this intrinsic ability to make you laugh out loud. Not only is he intelligently comical, but he also asks the most mind-blowing questions about the world. He sees and absorbs so much more detail than I do. Jack was diagnosed with Autism at three, and Hazel at six years old. You would never guess it when you first meet them. Particularly with Hazel – my little master of disguise…!

They are both verbal and love having a chat. When you are not observing them with a keen eye, they appear to be expressive children who make eye contact and naturally use gestures.

So much so that, when I first started to notice differences, educators instantly disagreed.

Autism in girls

Hazel was in Year One when we sought her diagnosis. Her class teacher was very fond of her and quite surprised when we raised it.

She instantly reassured us that Hazel was 'one of the children I don't need to worry about' and even mentioned that she happily sat at the back of the class. We really had to push for the school SENCO to be informed of our concerns and, when she was finally made aware, the SENCO's response was: 'I observed her for an hour, and I almost didn't see it but, just at the very end, I saw it. She is an expert masker!' Hazel appeared to be coping very well on the surface but there was so much hidden under a carefully created veneer. All it took was one hour of keen observation and a thorough understanding of how Autism presents in girls.

Hazel's class teacher was brilliant but simply unaware of how Autism presents in girls. Further training on the variety of presentation in girls would be immensely helpful for class teachers to ensure that others do not fall through the net.

Parent training

Jack had just turned three when he was diagnosed. At the time, we didn't fully understand Autism and were simply desperate for some guidance and support with our son's behaviour that was confusing and often disproportionate or difficult to explain. We threw ourselves into reading everything we could and started looking into Speech and Language Therapists (SLTs), ABA Therapists and Occupational Therapists (OTs). However, what made the single biggest difference for our family was attending parent courses. Being educated by SLTs and OTs about Autism instantly changed my understanding of Jack's needs and behaviours. His 'meltdowns' transformed into 'cries for help'. We adjusted how we spoke to him, how we prepared him for things, how we structured our home, and how we responded when he was distressed. That shift improved his regulation, our relationship, and his confidence far more quickly than we expected. Attending a parent training course was a powerful way to help support our child and it was also valuable to meet other parents and hear their experiences.

School environment

Like most parents, we are always keen to hear about ways to make our children's lives easier. We heard about another local school with a larger SEN department and decided to change schools. Jack would start Reception and Hazel would move into Year Two. We spent six months preparing for the change - lots of visits and time spent seeing the classrooms and meeting the teachers. Jack particularly built a bond with the SENCO and she was going to be the key bridge into the new environment. But just before the summer holidays, we found out that she was leaving and that there was no crossover with her replacement. In the first days of term, Jack appeared to cope but after a few days, the strain began to show and the school suggested he would need one-to-one support. We were surprised because he did not need this support in nursery. What we realise now is that Jack was not 'coping' - he was 'masking' in an unfamiliar place without the trusted adult he had prepared himself to rely on. The answer wasn't simply providing extra supervision through a one-to-one. The issue was that he didn't feel safe. We returned to his previous school, who worked thoughtfully to help him settle but even there, after a few weeks, the SENCO said to us, 'He is just so anxious in the classroom. I don't know if this environment is right for him at this time'. We decided to homeschool Jack for the near future and he is thriving with a full schedule of learning and activities. His anxiety levels have reduced, and he is much more regulated and happy. This taught us several things: the importance of trusted adults within the school, an open dialogue with parents of neurodivergent children about staffing changes, and the understanding that one-to-one support doesn't always fix the 'problem', particularly when the issue is anxiety and a child's sense of safety. I often feel like each of my children is their very own jigsaw puzzle and, as they grow and evolve, I need to find the next piece that helps me better understand them and support them.

Autism is not a label that defines them. It has been a lens that helps us and educators understand how to support them to thrive. Hazel and Jack are children whose needs are easy to miss unless you know how to look. When adults look differently, everything changes.

Parent story 3: Maeve Hoxha

There are so many layers of emotions and things I wished I had known earlier. Things I wish I hadn't preoccupied my time with, and not understanding myself and my emotions better at the start of the journey. While I am only writing a short passage, I think the best way of explaining life with an Autistic child is by writing some scenarios of my wonderful life with my son. And by sharing a few of these experiences with you, I hope it helps.

When my son was diagnosed with Autism I didn't know much about it. My son was nonspeaking, and I remember feeling very overwhelmed with it all trying to piece it all together and I would Google Autism and statistics late into the night to see if my son would ever speak and what the road ahead might look like. He was still so young and I was trying to figure it all out at once, feeling it would give me some control over the situation. I would constantly look at videos online when my son had gone to sleep, I was worrying, trying to make comparisons as if somehow this would predict my son's journey, his future and outcomes.

I remember thinking one evening this can't be helpful after Googling for the millionth time and looking at videos trying to draw comparison, trying to put time scales on things, looking at when other Autistic children had spoken. Upon reflection all this did was cause myself sleepless nights and anxiety and realistically you cannot draw comparisons as every child is unique and different just like every adult is.

Sometimes in the early stages of diagnosis all rationale goes out the window and what comes in is anxiety, worry and trying to understand Autism and the best way to help your child. My son was nonspeaking and I worried that he would never be able to communicate or be able to express himself, I worried about how he would cope in the world apart from all the other challenges he was facing. That's something that sat very heavy in my heart. I wish I had known now that Autistic children are so resilient and so powerful and that they find ways to communicate and they find ways to reach us. If I'd known what I know now I wouldn't have had so many restless nights.

If I give my advice to other parents, I would say only research things that are relevant to your child where they are now, learn what you can do to build skills and help them at their present stage. Do not overthink, do not try to predict, just be present in the moment your child is at.

The proverb 'How do you eat an elephant? One bite at a time' fits with this.

The approach is to focus on the current piece rather than the magnitude of the whole.

I'm also now a very strong believer in understanding our children's nervous system and helping them to be happy and regulated. At the beginning I was very fixated on milestones and education, I saw communication as only using words. I asked myself how could my child try to communicate and reach milestones if he was always dysregulated? In the early years I found focusing on helping my child to be regulated and happy helped with everything else.

I decided one night when at last a rational moment had kicked in that Googling all the time was not productive, so I stopped comparing .What I wanted and was seeking I realised was knowledge and helpful tips, advice and guidance. By educating myself with books and online courses that's when it completely changed for me. I then started to feel empowered in this journey and not just the overwhelming feeling of drowning at times.

Tips I would give parents:

- You cannot predict an Autistic child's development.
- Let go of preconceptions of what you thought parenthood would look like.
- Autistic children do have similarities of course to all children but they are more complex and individual in how they will approach their learning and goals.
- Sometimes it feels like they are overlooked in what they can achieve. There will be times in your journey when you just look over at them and think 'since when did you learn to do that?' and smile!
- It's letting go of our preconceptions of what we thought our children's childhood would look like. That's when we really start to understand and can advocate for our children. By changing the approach to my child and celebrating his individuality, this has made a huge difference.

- Never underestimate how deeply Autistic children do feel. Autistic children are very in tune with other people's as well as their own feelings. They feel so powerfully. They are very intuitive and highly receptive to other people's moods and feelings; it's an amazing ability that our children have and it's beautiful.

In the early stage after diagnosis my son was displaying more challenging behaviour and having lots of meltdowns. He was resistant to touch and very self-directed at times, he would bite himself if distressed and that would cause bruising and marks. He could not partake in activities children his own age could as this was so overwhelming for him. This part was very challenging and upsetting for me and him. Whilst some people are very kind we have encountered others who are not.

I have always believed in exposure, exposure and more exposure. It has not been easy, but I never gave up and I would say to other parents do not give up with trying new things. I wanted my son to be able to do things he loves and also try new things that I knew he would like. I took very small steps that didn't overwhelm and went at his pace. I didn't want the experience to have a negative impact on him as learnt memory is very important.

It's very hard at times, but I feel it is important to not stop exposing your child to different experiences that are within your child's limits and with gentle encouragement. I have found it is so very important to build small building blocks of skills to help my son in different situations throughout his life. When you have a bad experience it's very easy to want to retreat and not do it again but please do return just very slowly at the start. Each child is different but I did find by explaining very calmly, always at face level with my son that we were going to try something new, explaining his feelings were normal and going at his pace helped. This year for the first time we went to a Christmas show after three years of trying. This year to my absolute wonder and joy my son sat down and enjoyed the whole show.

Things that have helped in trying new things: I always found it helpful to take a bag of distractions that my son liked to help him feel relaxed and comfortable. When we try something new we always keep it short and sweet! I have found that leaving on a positive note before my son got dysregulated is important. I always made sure I paid close attention to my son's mood and when it was changing, I tuned in to what he needed. This built strong bonds between me and my son and gave him a feeling of being happy, secure and listened to. I found this helped as communication was and still is difficult for my son. My son is starting to use words and uses an Alternative and Augmentative Communication device, he is funny and likes communicating but we don't yet have a conversation with words, he is very good with pictures. I found that always showing my son that I understood his actions helped. This was our way of communicating: I would make the same sounds my son made when he was happy and then saying 'happy you're happy'. If my son made sounds I knew it meant he was anxious. I would get to eye level and say 'you're worried it's ok I'm here' and do something to soothe him. Communicating in this way has made a huge difference between me and my son; it was our way of talking with each other and my son feeling understood which made him feel in control.

I would say to anyone, either a parent or if you are working with a non-speaking child: try to recognise the different sounds and vocalisations they are making and let them know that you understand that these sounds represent different things. If they're happy, sad or anxious or excited it's a way of opening up communication for you both.

The trust that was built when he understood that I understood him gave him the confidence to be able to take part in things slowly. It also allowed my son to know that if he wasn't happy, I would be there to support him, or we would leave.

Sometimes things don't always go to plan and this can be hard. I remember one incident so very clearly: it was a hot summer's day and I thought taking my son to the zoo would be a lovely experience as it is a very typical outing for a child of his age to enjoy the zoo and engage. I was also trying to promote pointing and I thought this experience would help build skills with this. My son had not engaged around the zoo so I thought going on a safari truck would be an excellent idea. I was alone and we got on to the truck and I sat at the back as I normally do to try and give my son space so he doesn't get dysregulated or get sensory overload. I had also chosen a quieter time of the day to partake on the truck when it wouldn't be so busy but there were still other people on the truck. About a quarter of the way into the experience my son had a complete meltdown. He started to thrash and lash out and wanted to get off the truck, but we could not as we were now enclosed and had to go the whole way round. People were turning and looking and no assistance was offered, just disapproving looks and stares. My son then became so upset he started to pull my hair and was lashing out at me. I could feel the hard stares of others while I tried to calm my son. I knew there was no way of getting off the truck so I tried to remain calm and be as centred as I could. I just got on the floor with him so we were at eye level with each other. Being on his level calms my son, it's my way of saying 'I'm here buddy, I'm at your level, I'm right with you, I'm not leaving, I'm right here'. I spoke to him softly and with as few words as possible and stroked his arm which he always likes. I sat on the floor of the truck going round what seemed like eternity just sitting on the floor with my son laying on the bottom of the truck while I stroked him and my son was still screaming. By the time the truck stopped my son was now just rocking. When we got off no one assisted again. When we got back to the car and I had put my son safely into the car, he calmed down immediately like none of it had happened. I remember I closed the car door and turned away so he couldn't see me and I broke down. I remember crying, tears streaming down my face and just thinking, where does this leave us, will it always be like this, what can I do to help him, what have I done wrong as a mother? I also had another feeling, which now on reflection was completely irrational: it was shame. I can honestly say in that moment I felt broken for my son, for myself. I felt lost to what the future held and just in those few moments my world seemed to come crashing down on that hot summer's day. These moments will come from time to time and I will say it's ok to have hard days. I would say to any parent or educator, sit with your feelings and emotions, they are valid too. And I remember just wiping my eyes and then saying out loud, 'today will not end like this, we shall not end the day feeling like this'. We weren't far from the beach and my son loves to be free so we drove to the beach and when we arrived my son's whole body relaxed, as did my own, and he stripped off his clothes and he just ran on that beach and he laughed and he splashed in the waves, rolled in the sand, all his senses became alive but with positive feelings, the hours before fading away replaced with sheer joy. I decided that our journey wasn't the typical journey but in fact a new path was to be taken. And while we still had dreams and goals they were to be achieved differently. Every child is different, and every child is unique.

I would say try to create a life with opportunities by doing things that your child will enjoy. I learned to remove pressures from my son very early on. By giving my son freedom he is more regulated and is able to learn skills in these moments.

If I could give any advice to a parent starting out or someone who is still unsure (I'm still figuring it out myself and learning every day) it would be this: do not waste time on trying to piece everything together because our children are complex and wonderful and forever evolving and changing at their own rhythm. Let go of preconceptions. Celebrate their small triumphs as loudly as possible and take real joy in those small steps because looking back those very small steps that I had championed so loudly were actually the small building blocks to some of the bigger goals my son now achieves and it was in all those small pieces a beautiful jigsaw was coming together very slowly. It's far from finished but it is good to look how far you have come.

Learn to regulate yourself and your feelings and anxieties because to our children we are their centre and we have to be strong within our role and it is very difficult in the beginning but please do not burn out because your children need you to be as whole as possible.

I know that is difficult but please make time for yourself even if it's a quiet hour at the end of the day to reflect on how well you have done as well. I now take the bad days as windows of opportunity to learn about my son. I ask myself why was that day harder? What upset him? What dysregulated him? What tools can I give him to communicate better with me that he didn't want to do something or was finding it too stressful?

If we have a bad day or moment I make sure that it is replaced by something happy even if it's putting on the music and dancing or tickling; anything to lift my son's spirits again. It's very important for our children to feel secure and happy and understood. Don't Google to compare, Google to research activities and training you can do online and things that promote self-awareness and help advocate for our children. Every child is completely individual so just be led by your child and develop skills and experiences that expose your children to new things. Being by their side is an enriching part of parenting an Autistic child.

I see my son's life with Autism as a very complex beautiful jigsaw and each piece is slowly being put together to make this most magnificent jigsaw. It's vibrant, it's colourful, it has depth, hidden pieces, it's intricate, it can be frustrating, it can be overwhelming, but when the pieces start to come together it's the most beautiful and rewarding feeling and joyful thing to see.

Parent story 4

Our initial concerns about our daughter, namely being easily upset, difficult to settle and a terrible sleeper, were largely ignored by health professionals. At appointments, they were amazed by her early speech, singing, reciting the planets/seasons, counting and problem solving abilities. On taking her to a paediatrician, their only concern was that she might be 'a bit too clever'. When our daughter was showing no interest in any ball games at age 2.5yrs, I took her to see a private physiotherapist who raised concerns that she may be Autistic.

From that point, we waited nearly 2 years before being offered an Autism assessment through the NHS. In the meantime, our daughter had started nursery and her difficulties had become significantly more pronounced. We therefore sought a private diagnosis as we felt it was needed to both assist nursery staff supporting her and also to enable open discussions with future schools.

In my experience, in South London, we have received no support from the NHS. Despite my daughter's anxiety and meltdowns limiting us accessing the community and opportunities required for her development, when I requested a CAMHS referral, I was told there was no point as she would not meet the threshold. With much persuasion, a paediatrician agreed to make a referral to Speech and Language Therapy, but they never made contact.

For us, accessing support has been a vastly bigger challenge than getting a diagnosis. In the context of not being able to access support via the NHS, we have relied upon the private sector. Over the years, we have seen many private practitioners, some of whom have changed our lives for the better, and some who have undoubtedly been detrimental to our daughter and us as parents.

In our experience, seeking advice from a Speech and Language Therapist who specialises in young children with Autism was key in identifying strategies that were appropriate and achievable. We have also found Occupational Therapists and Psychologists to be a source of support, if financial resources allow for input from additional professionals.

We have found educators, and ourselves at times, to be, understandably, focused on changing our daughter's challenging behaviours and increasing her compliance with what we wanted/needed her to do. Three years into our journey, I am now of the view that children this age aren't really able to change themselves or their behaviours. The interventions which reduced her challenging behaviours, and increased her compliance, were working with adults to modify the environment and their expectations of our daughter, and supporting her to feel less anxious.

In our experience, professionals who focused primarily on stopping her engaging in challenging behaviours caused our daughter to become extremely distressed and more anxious, with an increase in challenging behaviours. Initially we thought that, as experts, they must know what they are doing and that we would be letting our daughter down by not staying the course with these interventions. We now bitterly regret having exposed our daughter to that, and fear they will have had a lasting impact on her self-esteem and trust in us.

As our daughter has gotten older, and her communication has improved, the 'gaps' in her skills/knowledge have become easier to identify. When she was 5 years old and another mum put a bag of duck food out, to offer my daughter to take some, I realised she didn't understand basic gestures. On her asking me why I was angry when I was concentrating or confused, I came to realise that she struggles to read facial expressions. On repeatedly becoming distressed when hearing people use the word 'really' to indicate surprise or doubt (as opposed to 'really fast' or 'really big'), I came to realise that her understanding of language is very concrete, to the extent that significant proportions of conversation are incomprehensible to her. With this in mind, I have come to appreciate her profound lack of understanding about what was going on, when she was in nursery, and how anxiety provoking that must have been.

I think our daughter's strong intellectual abilities, like reading fluently and her impressive vocabulary, left educators, and myself, underestimating the extent of the gaps in her skills/knowledge. The brilliant thing about identifying those gaps has been that we've been able to teach our daughter to 'plug the gaps', she has become less anxious and her challenging behaviours have reduced. But it has taken her maturing for us to be able to identify these nuanced triggers.

Our experience of the early years system has been difficult. Although we had concerns prior to our daughter starting nursery, her difficulties became much more pronounced in the nursery environment. The obvious way to access help is via an EHCP. However, since starting the initial EHCP application, it took nearly 2.5 years for our daughter to get an EHCP, by which time she had already started school. As such, the practical support available to the nursery was solely what we, as parents, could provide the nursery with. Despite privately funding a Teaching Assistant, Speech and Language Therapist and Occupational Therapy sessions, our daughter's ability to cope in the nursery setting was varied. We eventually came to the conclusion that our daughter should be in education for however many hours were beneficial for her. And that any hours beyond that were detrimental. As such, at times, we reduced the number of hours/day, reduced the number of days at nursery (getting a home tutor for the days not at nursery) and took her out of nursery for several weeks at one point where her anxiety and behaviours indicated to us that she needed a complete break to recover.

The educational provision which was offered to us by the local authority was not, in our opinion, appropriate for our daughter's profile. We have therefore been left in the vulnerable position of relying on private nurseries and schools, where we have felt that we have had to accept sometimes terrible treatment, for fear of our daughter being expelled and being forced into what the local authority have stipulated. At one point, the nursery hired our private Teaching Assistant for a different role in their school, without giving us any warning, so our daughter was unable to attend the nursery whilst we sought a replacement. They then had a change of head and we were told, at short notice, that our daughter would not be allowed to stay for the following year which left us scrambling to identify a suitable school.

We have found parenting an Autistic child to be a lonely and isolating experience. We have frequently felt judged, and at times blamed, for our daughter's challenging behaviours and have subsequently avoided accessing a range of places in the community. Whilst at nursery, we stopped taking our daughter to birthday parties, because they were overwhelming, and she was consistently having meltdowns. We were doing drop offs and pickups at different times to other parents, so we rarely met them. Transitions are challenging so we would avoid pausing to chat for fear of derailing them. I even removed myself from the parent WhatsApp groups, as reading other parents' messages about their concerns about there not being enough forest school or what to take to the bake sale emphasised how much bigger our problems were and how different our lives were from families with neurotypical children.

I think it is hard for people to comprehend the extent to which having an Autistic nursery-age child took over all aspects of our lives: from the practical aspects of being unable to access lots of places which are part of normal family life, effectively only having access to very small hours of childcare, the stress of identifying appropriate schools and the burden of instituting the advice of professionals, to the considerable financial and administrative asks. We have had to self-fund Teaching Assistants and therapies, effectively become an HR department recruiting, writing contracts for and paying TAs and home schoolteachers, and in pursuing the EHCP processing (which has involved working with lawyers, barristers and our local MP). Latterly I had to give up my job as there was simply not the capacity for us both to be working. This has predictably added further financial strain. I am somewhat ashamed to admit that my own reaction to the news that my daughter was likely Autistic was in-keeping with a grief reaction, for the loss of the future life we assumed our daughter (and our family) would have, and accepting the reality that she may never live an independent life.

Tips for parents with nursery-age children:

- It's much easier said than done, but try not to catastrophise over 'missed milestones'. Toileting and writing were huge struggles for us and the more the adults around our daughter were anxious about these, the more avoidant our daughter became to even attempt them. Shifting the focus on our daughter being happy and relaxed and taking things slowly, was much more conducive to making strides in her development. We got there in the end but on our daughter's timetable which is ok.
- Challenging behaviours can be so shaming for parents. Try not to focus too much on eliminating the behaviour. Instead, be a detective and focus on identifying the 'gaps' and plugging them. In our experience, identifying the subtle 'gaps' got much easier with age. Be realistic about when you will see improvements. Building up skills takes time. There is no magic wand (and people who offer one should be avoided).
- We have found preparation for new experiences using social stories (from the big things like starting nursery to the seemingly small changes in routine) to be very helpful in reducing anxiety. Using photographs of the people you will meet and the place you are going can be immensely helpful.
- In a world of appointments with professionals and concerns from nursery, there have been many conversations about our daughter's difficulties. It is still surprising to me how many people initiate those conversations in front of our daughter. Our daughter is highly intelligent and very sensitive and repeatedly being witness to these conversations is clearly detrimental to her self-esteem. To avoid this, we as parents now request a phone call with professionals to answer any questions before taking our daughter to appointments. Similarly, we have proactively had to ask nursery/school staff to ensure discussions about incidents are not being had at the school gates.
- Obtaining an EHCP for our daughter has been a very challenging process. Be prepared for a long fight and invest in getting a good lawyer if you possibly can.
- Having a nursery-age Autistic child is uniquely challenging and has, at times, felt like we are fighting multiple fronts. Identifying an ally who has practical experience in the field, in our case a Speech and Language Therapist, has been key for navigating the system, being a source of emotional support and a sounding board for us in times of having to make difficult decisions we have felt wholly unqualified to make.

Understanding the full picture – being a detective

Now that you have taken time to read and digest theories, key concepts and parental perspectives we are going to look at how you can pull this knowledge together to understand the full picture whilst keeping in mind that every child and family are different. This is a helpful next step before we move onto strategies and practical tools. It is vital that we take the time to understand the full picture for each child. Often, I will hear well-meaning comments like 'we have had lots of Autistic children, we know what to do'. Whilst it is great to hear of experience, it is also very important to recognise individual differences and the fact that not every Autistic child will present the same way and may in fact need very different support.

In my work I often spend time talking to parents and educators about detective work; about really taking time to step back to understand what is going on for an individual child. Sometimes this detective work is done by several professionals, such as an occupational therapist, SLT and clinical psychologist, but at other times this level of support is not available. In simple terms, doing detective work means 'getting in the shoes' of the children we work with to understand how they experience the world. There are lots of different ways to do this, but one helpful way is through using the iceberg model (see Figure 2.1). We use this model in more detail in Chapter 7 when

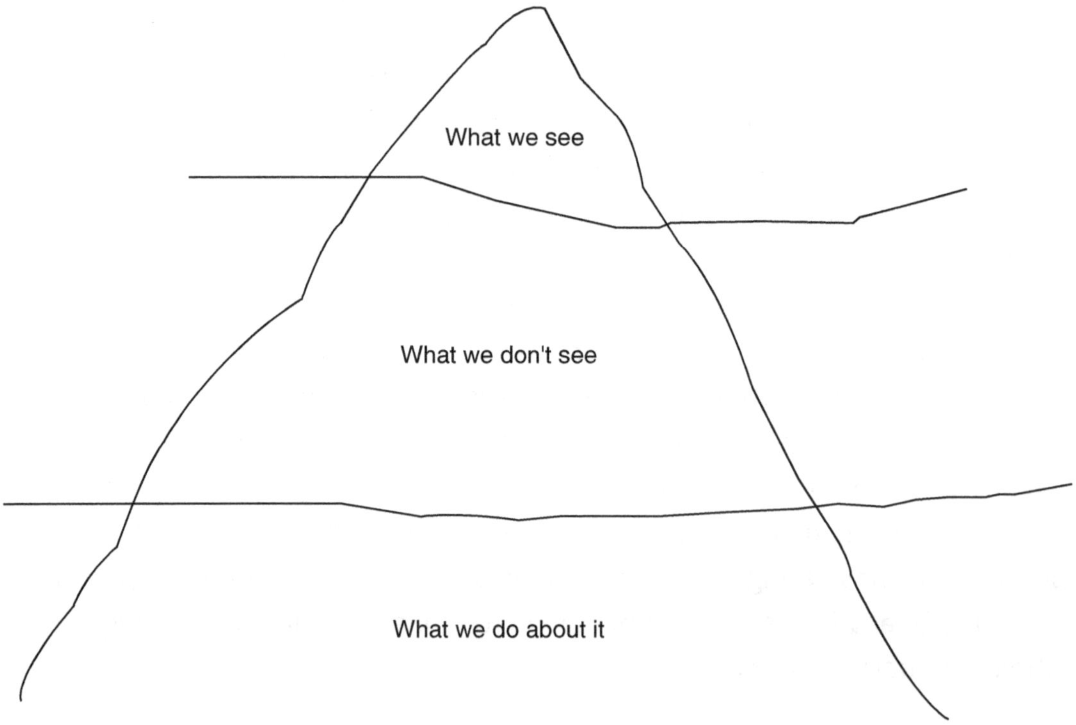

Figure 2.1 The iceberg model

we think specifically about behaviour. However, I think it is a really helpful tool to understand Autism in terms of what is seen and what is unseen. In simple terms, what we see at the surface is only the 'tip of the iceberg'. If we look under the water line and explore what is unseen, we can understand more about 'why' something may be occurring. Without understanding the 'why' we don't have a good rationale for support and intervention. It can be easy to jump from the 'what we see part' on the surface to 'what we do about it' without considering the parts that we don't see. We can use the iceberg to think about individual strengths and differences and as a way to zoom out from a situation, to gather more knowledge and to get in the child's shoes. Without this knowledge, collaborative problem solving and effective strategies are less likely.

Let's do an iceberg in relation to Louie who we talked about in Chapter 1 (see page 22). Remember we talked about Louie loving water play. We can think about what we see and what is the unseen part which can help us to problem solve what we need to do (see Figure 2.2).

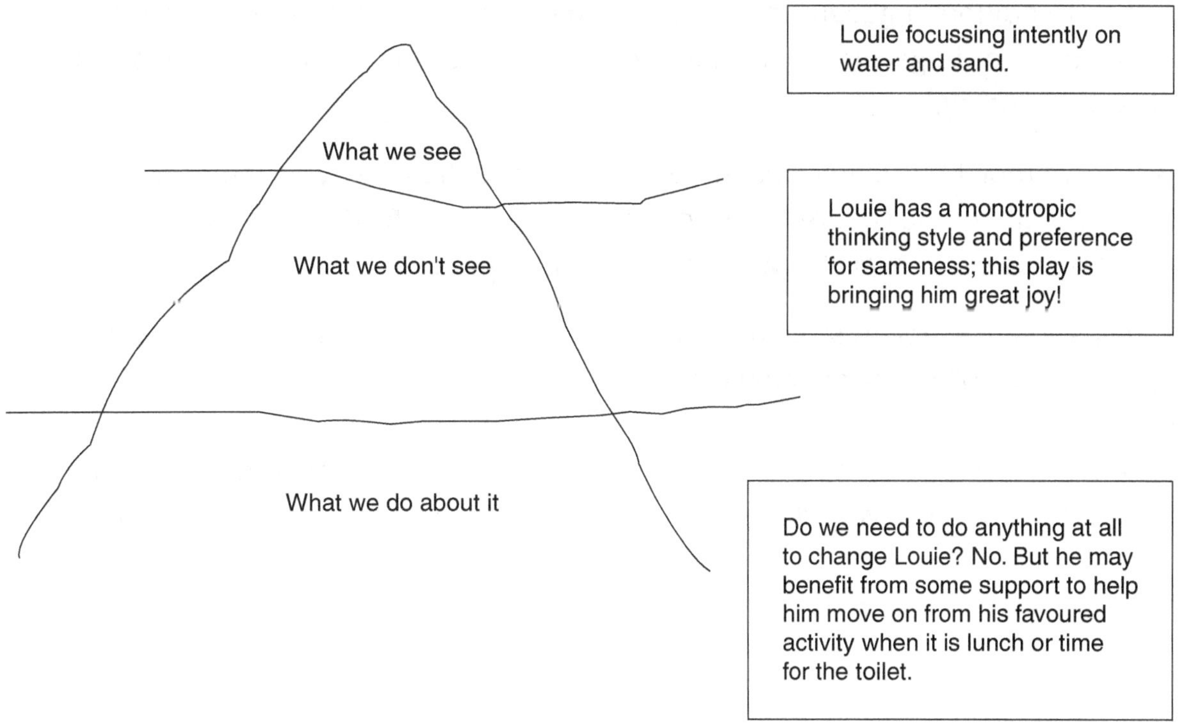

Figure 2.2 Louie's iceberg

Activity

Think of a child that you work with. Draw out an iceberg and think about what may be going on underneath the waterline.

Let's get started!

Now that you have a good understanding of Autism and Autistic thinking styles, let's get started in using this manual. This manual provides several different tools to help you learn more about the children in your setting. These tools are designed to help you make observations and gather relevant information to help support and problem solve.

Support for Autistic children can be a post code lottery and may vary hugely depending on your area, which was highlighted in the parent stories earlier in this chapter. In reality, this means that some children start an education environment with a diagnosis and support in place, whereas other children may start without a diagnosis or referral to any relevant professionals. This can feel very overwhelming for both parents and staff in the setting. A helpful starting point is through gathering information and observations which can be helpful when it comes to referral for an assessment or for applying for an EHCP. Whilst different geographical areas tend to have certain ways to write individual learning plans or targets it is still helpful to use the following tools to build observations and understanding.

The Iceberg tool (I:1) and Information-Gathering sheet (I:2) help you gather relevant information about the children you work with. See pages 45–46 for blank copies for you to copy and use; also available with online support materials.

(I:1) helps you to problem solve what may be 'unseen' or going on below the waterline. (I:2) is a way to collect observations. (I:2) is aimed to be used for a specific activity, e.g. a child may have one completed at lunch time or break time and then another at a different time. Observing a child in the moment and taking lots of notes is much more helpful than retrospectively filling in an observation form that is aimed at the full day.

I:1 The Iceberg tool: Use the iceberg to problem solve

I:1

What we see:

What is going on under the surface:

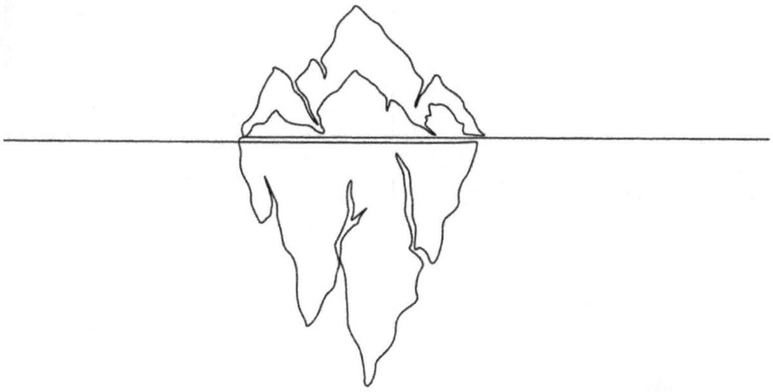

Figure 2.3

I:2 Information gathering tool

I:2

Name:	
DOB:	
Date and context of observation:	
Communication: include observations of all forms of communication and a language sample if relevant. Include different functions of communication including requesting, commenting, protests, questions.	
Understanding: - Routines - Key words - Instructions - Transitions	
Sensory preferences: Include sensitivities as well as likes and dislikes.	
Play and interests: What does the child spend time doing, what are they enjoying?	
Social relationships: Who is important and what does the child like to do?	
Strengths observed:	
Barriers: Think about what is making life hard for a child.	
Other observations:	

Chapter 2 summary

- Listening and working in collaboration is important. Words matter, the parent perspectives in this chapter highlight the role we have in supporting parents on their journey and the challenges many parents face in accessing the support that their child needs.
- The iceberg is a helpful tool to use to understand what may be going on for a child. We can use this to build understanding rather than jumping to conclusions. There is always more than what we see at the surface.
- Be curious and try to look below the waterline! Use the iceberg to think about what may be going on for children that you work with.

3

The early years environment

Barriers and support

Chapter 3 provides the following:

- Consideration of barriers in the early years environment for Autistic children
- Overview of reasonable adjustments
- Tools and strategies to change the environment to make it more accessible for Autistic children
- Relevant frameworks and approaches
- What it is like working with an occupational therapist
- Strategies on how we can increase understanding in the early years environment through use of visual supports, routines and structured teaching
- Activity sheets:
  (E:1) – Using objects to support understanding
  (E:2) – Using photos to help understanding
  (E:3) – Using a first/then board
  (E:4) – Understanding the concept 'finished' and using a countdown
  (E:5) – Using a visual timetable
  (E:6) – Understanding the concept of 'wait' and using a wait card
  (E:7) – Using visuals to support taking part in everyday activities
  (E:8) – Language for routines
  (E:9) – Structuring the learning environment – let's make a plan
  (E:10) – Structuring the learning environment – top tips
  (E:11) – Structuring a one-on-one area using a workstation
  (E:12) – Structuring one-on-one activities
  (E:13) – Supporting changes in the routine
  (E:14) – Using social stories
  (E:15) – Strategy sheet template

DOI: 10.4324/9781003627760-3

Early years education

Starting in education can be a daunting prospect for all parents and their children. These feelings may be amplified for a parent of an Autistic child. The parent stories in Chapter 2 highlighted both strengths and barriers within education and how these can have a huge impact on a parent and their child. Whilst early years education is important and can be incredibly supportive, for some Autistic children the environment itself can be stressful and overwhelming. New people, sounds, smells, routines and unclear expectations can all be huge barriers to overcome. Some early years environments are highly structured and others are free flow; both can present barriers for Autistic children. When we think about early years environments it is important to acknowledge that for some children a nursery environment isn't the right environment to support them and in fact can do more harm.

We need to work hard on changing the environment and putting adjustments in place for Autistic children. Working with parents and collaborating closely is a key first step in thinking about how best to support each individual child within the environment.

From your reading of relevant theories and key concepts in Chapter 1 you can start to think about some of the barriers that Autistic children may face in an early years education environment. Acknowledging these barriers and being flexible in our approach to adjusting is an important first step.

Activity

Think about your environment. Are there any barriers that may make it hard for an Autistic child to access parts of the day or routine? Think about different elements of the environment and what these look like in your setting (e.g. the physical environment, structure of the day, sensory impact, social environment and approach to learning).

In Chapter 1 we talked about Dr. Luke Beardon's (2017) framework of Autism + Environment = Outcome and in Chapter 2 we visited parental stories that highlighted how the environment has a huge impact on an Autistic child. A key message to take away from this chapter is how important it is that we 'change the environment'. As a starting point to making the environment accessible it is important to think about reasonable adjustments in early years.

Reasonable adjustments

Reasonable adjustments are important as they help children feel safe and ready to learn. They come from the Equality Act (2010); in simple terms a reasonable adjustment means a legal duty to change things so that an Autistic person is not put at a disadvantage. This means removing barriers that are in the environment, rather than thinking that the child needs to change to fit the environment. The legal duty applies to early years settings and nurseries, so it is important to have an awareness of what reasonable adjustments entail as they are important in reducing barriers and making the early years environment accessible. It is also important to note that the legal duty exists even if a child does not yet have a diagnosis. This is because Autism is considered a disability in law. I have found access to reasonable adjustments in early years and schools can vary hugely as there is often a lack of understanding around what can be done in the environment. It is important to emphasise that reasonable adjustments are not dependent on having a diagnosis, something a parent or a child needs to earn, a special favour or rewards for behaviour. They are a legal right. These things may seem obvious but sadly and all too often I have seen practitioners and educators who hold these outdated views and see these vital adaptations as 'special treatments'.

Getting to know a child and understanding what reasonable adjustments they need is a key step in making the environment accessible and overcoming barriers.

Table 3.1 summarises some example reasonable adjustments for the early years environment. This is just a starting point. Think about what reasonable adjustments are important for the children you work with.

I would encourage you to consider what each individual Autistic child needs in terms of reasonable adjustments and write them up in conjunction with parents.

Supporting success

Ensuring that the start to an education environment is successful can have a huge impact on a child, the family and also the staff working with the child. The good news is there is lots that can be done to support an Autistic child before starting at nursery to ensure that the environment is supportive to their needs. Preparation, understanding and good communication are key factors in supporting success in the early years. Some of the most successful placements and transitions for Autistic children I have seen have hinged on these key principles. In many cases these have been in early years settings with limited prior experience of Autism. However, a willingness and commitment to learn and listen makes all the difference.

Table 3.1 Examples of reasonable adjustments in early years

Summary of reasonable adjustments guiding principle: adjust the environment and expectations not the child	
Create predictability and structure	- Use of visual timetables (photos or symbols) and first/then boards - A consistent adult as a key person for child and parents - Warning around when key adults are away or there are changes in the routine
Sensory	- Access to quiet spaces and low arousal areas if needed - Reduced regulations around any uniform or clothing - Adaptations to mealtimes and food available, e.g. a child is allowed to bring in their own food
Transitions and routines	- Extra time to settle in the morning - Staggered starting times to avoid busy and overwhelming drop offs and pick-ups - Reduced timetable with more flexible attendance and shorter sessions - Allowing transitional objects from home
Communication	- Use clear, direct language - Avoid ambiguity and implied meanings - Give processing time - Use total communication approaches - Accept that all forms of communication are valid - Recognise that behaviour is often an attempt to communicate
Play and learning	- Follow a child's interests - Understand the role of monotropism - Give access to special interests - Remember that play and interaction look different - Give breaks that are meaningful - Don't force group play or sharing
Emotion regulation support	- Recognise early signs of overwhelm, be a detective and communicate with parents - Provide a trusted adult to support co-regulation - Talk to parents about masking and holding it together - Avoid punitive responses to distress
Behaviour	- Reduce demands - Recognise meltdowns and shutdowns are different from tantrums - Focus on safety and wellbeing
Working with parents and carers	- Share observations not judgements - Don't talk about a child in front of them - Communicate changes in advance

Tip

In my work as an SLT I have been lucky to work with wonderful educators and health-care professionals. Some of the key principles emphasised by these wonderful people have stuck with me and can be top tips for anyone working with Autistic children.

Keeping these in your mind as guiding principles can be a useful starting point when we think about environmental changes and strategies.

- Change yourself ... not the child.
- Adjust the environment, make sure reasonable adjustments are in place and everyone knows what they are.
- Adjust your expectations of a child. Ask yourself what is functional, realistic and supportive.
- Work as a team. Ensure that everyone knows the strategies for a particular child rather than it being left to one person.
- Show me, don't tell me. Use visuals wherever possible to support Autistic children's strength in visual processing.
- Always start with strengths.
- Bring structure to the unstructured.
- Be prepared – think in advance what a child will need (this takes time and planning).
- Give strategies time to work. I have worked within settings that have implemented changes to the environment and then discarded them after they haven't worked after a week. Think how long it takes to change any behaviour in an adult or a child; make sure that you give enough time (at least a half term) to allow for change.
- Listen and work collaboratively.

Working with an occupational therapist (OT): supporting Autistic children to develop skills needed for everyday tasks

SLTs and OTs often work in conjunction with each other to support children in their daily environments. I have asked my OT colleague Annmarie Sims to outline the role of the OT in supporting Autistic children:

> The role of the OT is to help children participate in all the activities that 'occupy' their day. That is why we are called OTs. For young children the focus is often on developing self-care skills such as using the toilet, dressing, brushing teeth, washing, participating at mealtimes and sleep – an activity that takes up many hours of the day. Another important occupation of childhood is play, both playing alone (self-occupation) and playing with others. Participating at school (learning) and participating in family life also occupy children's lives.

This book is about helping Autistic children with communication in the early years. Hence a section on developing the child's ability to participate in daily occupations is appropriate as teaching and guiding a child through their day and all the activities that involves cannot be done without communication. The adult communicates an instruction, and the child communicates a response. The child may communicate through their behaviour to demonstrate they are unsure of what is expected, unsure how to do it or that the task the adult is wanting them to do is not of interest or meaningful and they would rather occupy themselves in another way. It is therefore important for the OT and the speech and language therapist to work closely together to support the child to participate in daily life.

OT Assessment

An OT will ask you lots of questions about the daily routine. We want to understand your lived experience to help problem solve challenges with participation and with completing daily activities.

Questions about all the different areas of your child's development and the impact on their occupations

- Learning skills – problem solving, remembering information, how is the child learning at nursery?
- Motor skills – both big movements (gross motor skills) and hand skills (fine motor skills).
- Sensory responses – sensory experiences your child likes and those they dislike (for example they may like soft clothes and dislike sudden noises or strong smells). They may not feel the cold or pain, or they may be very sensitive.
- Social interaction skills and social interest.
- What are their interests? What do they like to play with?
- And communication skills – understanding what others communicate and how they communicate with others.

Questions about the environment where the activity happens

- Who else is present and what is their relationship to the child?
- The physical and sensory environment – for example noise, lights and smells as well as physical setup of the environment.

- The unique cultural environment as everyone has different customs, daily routines and beliefs.

Questions about the occupation that you would like help with

- The OT will ask questions about how your child participates in daily activities. Here are some examples:
  - Does your child understand and follow the routine of getting dressed, do they extend their arms and legs through the clothes? Do they have strong preferences for how the clothes feels?
  - If toileting is a skill your child needs help with the OT will want to know if the child is aware when they need to open their bowels or if they know what the toilet is for? The OT will help you with where to start.
  - Brushing teeth – is it the taste of the toothpaste or feel of the toothbrush your child struggles with? How is the task done?
- It is not possible to list all the occupations that the child may find challenging, these are just examples. Speak to your OT about your concerns

Just like strategies to support sleep are practised when it is time to sleep, dressing, eating, playing and toileting, etc., should be supported at the right time and in the environment, where the task naturally occurs, such as home or nursery. For example, practising dressing skills when it is time to get dressed will make much more sense to your child than if practised at another time of day. Skills should also be practised when there is time to do so, so maybe start with pyjamas rather than school uniform during a hectic morning routine.

The OT will help you to understand why the child is struggling with a particular occupation and will suggest strategies to help your child to participate and develop their skills. It is important adults do not assume what the barriers are or that they lie solely within the child. By recognising the interplay between the child, the environment and the task, the OT will help to adapt the environment and the task and develop your child's skills to help them succeed with daily occupations.

Using visual supports and a total communication approach to support access to the environment

Communication is much more than just spoken words and all forms of communication are valid. A total communication approach emphasises not just spoken words; it embraces all forms of communication so that Autistic children can understand and be understood.

In this chapter we are focussing on supporting an Autistic child's ability to understand so that they can have access to the environment. We can make the environment more accessible through total communication and making our own communication more visual.

'*Show me don't just tell me*' is a mantra many SLTs and specialist teachers live by. Spoken words are transient and for many children are missed. If you can show children what is happening visually as well as using gestures, visuals and spoken words, their understanding is supported. Many interventions for Autistic children use visuals as a key part. It makes sense to use a child's strengths as a starting point and we know that Autistic children have strengths in their visual processing.

What are visual supports?

Firstly, it is helpful to clarify the difference in using visuals to help a child understand and using visuals to support expressive communication. I have visited many settings where all visual supports have been referred to as 'PECS'. PECS stands for the picture exchange communication system and is an alternative and augmentative system developed in 1985 in the United States. SLTs don't really use PECS anymore and there are lots of better and more affirmative ways to support spoken communication (more on this in Chapter 4). However, I still hear lots of people using the word PECS. I would encourage you to replace this term with 'visual supports'. Visual supports can be useful to help a child make a request or a choice or send you a message (expressive communication). We also use visual supports to help understanding (receptive communication), for example, a timetable, first/then board or photographs. This chapter focusses on using visual supports for understanding.

Visual supports can be objects, pictures, photos and miniature objects. The key part is that they are permanent, unlike a spoken word or gesture which once spoken or signed disappears. Using visual supports provides extra information alongside the spoken word to help a child understand. I have found there is the added extra that using the visual support tends to slow down an adult's talking which will also naturally help a child's understanding of language.

We all use visual supports in our daily lives to help us complete tasks and understand information. Think of your to-do list or cooking something new from a recipe book or imagine being in a foreign country where you may find it hard to understand and speak the language. You would likely be reliant on visual cues around you to help you understand; you might point to a map or sign or show a picture in your guidebook. These are all similar to using visuals to support communication.

It is important to be aware that some visual supports are easier to understand than others. Whether to use an object, picture or symbol should depend on each individual child's learning style and understanding. Objects are generally viewed as the easiest to understand. A child's ability to understand visuals relates to their developmental stage and is known as symbolic representation. The more concrete the visual support, the easier it is to understand; for example, showing a nappy each time a child is going to be changed is easier to comprehend than looking at a picture of a nappy. The hierarchy of symbolic representation from easiest to hardest to understand is shown in Figure 3.1. It is useful to bear this in mind as all too often we start using symbols when actually a child may not be ready for these.

Tip

- Avoid images such as cartoons and those that you may find on clip art. These can be confusing for children.
- Recognise that different children may need different visuals depending on their individual profile. For example, in the same setting one child may require objects of reference and another may use a written checklist with a whiteboard and a pen.

Ensure that any visuals used at home are the same as those in the education setting. It could be confusing for a child to have different systems at home and nursery. One of the most portable and easily accessible ways to provide visuals (if a child is able to understand line drawings) is to use a wipe-clean whiteboard and draw the visual

Easiest to Understand

REAL OBJECT
MINIATURE OBJECT
PHOTOGRAPH
LINE DRAWING
SYMBOL
↓ WRITTEN WORD

Hardest to Understand

Figure 3.1 Hierarchy of symbolic representation

supports. This has the added bonus of being portable and easy for parents to also use so there is continuity between the education environment and home.

Turn now to the following activity sheets (pages 64–77) for practical ideas on supporting understanding in a visual way:

(E:1) – Using objects to support understanding
(E:2) – Using photos to help understanding
(E:3) – Using a first/then board
(E:4) – Understanding the concept 'finished' and using a countdown
(E:5) – Using a visual timetable
(E:6) – Understanding the concept of 'wait' and using a wait card
(E:7) – Using visuals to support taking part in everyday activities

Activity

Think of an Autistic child who would benefit from one of the visual supports outlined here (E:1)–(E:7). Plan how you would implement the resource into your setting.

Consider the following:

- In what way will this support the child?
- What do you hope will be different after introducing the visual support?
- How will you put the strategy in place?
- How will you ensure consistency?

Alex is three and a half; he is Autistic. He is able to understand short instructions and communicates using short sentences. He loves playing with trains and doesn't want to do anything else at nursery. Recently staff working with him have noticed that he has started to be interested in the sand area when his trains are not visible, he really enjoys being with the other children at the sand tray and adults are keen to give him opportunities to engage in new activities that he will enjoy. Alex can become upset when trains are finished and when he needs to transition onto any other activity.

Table 3.2 Strategy planning sheet: example

Child's name:	*Alex*
Aim: Rationale:	For Alex to transition between activities without distress. • To support understanding and predictability • Reduce anxiety and overwhelm • Free up energy for play and learning
Strategy/activity to be introduced:	Using a first/then board (E:3) Understanding the concept 'finished' and using a countdown (E:4)
How this will help:	The first/then board will help Alex understand what is happening next and transition between activities. Staff will encourage Alex to engage in a different activity (that he also enjoys) and then have the trains which are predictable and familiar to him, e.g. first sand then trains.
What will be different for Alex:	Increased joy and enjoyment in activities. Less stress when trains finish as the world will feel more predictable.
How to implement:	• Strategy to be discussed at staff meeting to ensure consistency • Strategy planning sheet to be shared with staff (E:15)

See printable (E:15) for strategy planning street.

Staff working with Alex would like him to engage in other activities and to transition between activities with less upset; they have identified that he will benefit from the use of a first/then board (E:3) and countdown (E:4).

Use of routines

We can effectively use routines to help children understand their environment. Routines are brilliant as we tend to do them every day, they are familiar and can be very comforting. In Chapter 1 we learnt that predictability and consistency of routines can be very comforting and supportive to Autistic children. Many parents of Autistic children tell me that their children thrive on predictability and learn well through routines. Really, when you think about it, we all learn well, especially when it is new information, in a routine and predictable way. Routines and consistency can make it easier for Autistic children to understand what is happening throughout the day. This can in turn help reduce anxiety. Routines can be comforting and supportive to learning. We can build visual supports, consistent language and songs into our everyday routines to make them more predictable for Autistic children.

- The great thing about routines is that they happen throughout the day so can be a natural way to build in consistent language and learning opportunities.
- You can support a child's understanding in everyday routine activities like hand washing or getting ready for lunch or nap time; this has the added advantage

of not feeling like you have to make 'separate time' to work on communication targets.

- Building these key strategies into your routines can have a big impact on the children who you are working with.
- I am often so impressed with the families I work with who take simple strategies and incorporate them into routine activities across the day. This then becomes part of the routine so that the strategies you are using just become automatic rather than being seen as something that is separate and extra to do.
- Turn now to activity sheet (E:8) 'Language for routines' for strategies that you can incorporate into your everyday routines.

Let's look at Jack to see how staff working with him used routines and visuals to help him overcome some of the barriers in the environment. This made things more predictable for him.

Case study: supporting Jack's understanding

Background

Jack started nursery at age two and a half; at this time, he was non-speaking and did not tend to respond when others spoke to him. When he started nursery, he became upset whenever an adult attempted to direct him onto an activity or take him to change his nappy or wash his hands and would only engage with cars lying down watching them at eye level. He didn't participate in the routines of the nursery and was generally self-directed. Staff working with him were keen to help him engage more so that he could access new and different learning opportunities. Jack found it hard to ask for things that he wanted. He would communicate by screaming and pushing items away to show that he didn't want something. He occasionally took an adult's hand to lead to the area he wanted something and would reach towards a preferred item. Often Jack would climb to reach what he wanted and became frustrated when unable to communicate.

Actions

Staff got to know Jack and used the iceberg model to think about what was going on for him. This was a helpful step in problem solving what may be helpful. They considered that the environment was probably very stressful and overwhelming for

Jack. They completed the Information-Gathering sheet (I:2; see page 46) and talked through their observations with parents. From this they were able to identify his profile of strengths and needs. Staff met with Jack's parents to discuss targets. Parents and staff agreed on the following targets (to support Jack's understanding):

Targets

- For Jack to understand the routine of the nursery with visual supports
- For staff to help Jack to understand the concept finished

Strategies used

Over Jack's first six months staff used the following strategies:

- They consistently used objects to support his understanding (see E:1).
- As a staff group, they focussed on using consistent language – as outlined in (E:8). At a staff meeting they discussed this and realised how much inconsistency there was between them, for example, some people saying 'time for toilet', others saying 'nappy time' and so on.
- They consistently used strategies around helping Jack understand the concept of 'finished' (see E:4).
- This particular group of staff were quite musical and decided to introduce a routine song for different activities including tidy up, snack time, shoes on/off, as well as showing an object to support understanding.

The results

Jack is understanding more and is less stressed by the environment. He is now able to respond to cues; for example, when shown a nappy he will now walk towards the change station, and when shown the object for outside he will walk towards the door. One of the major benefits is that he is calm and not becoming distressed in the same way which is important to his wellbeing. Although it was not a goal, staff have noticed that Jack plays less with the cars and is happy to explore a range of activities. Jack has started to hum the tidy-up song at home.

We will revisit Jack in Chapter Four to look at how staff targeted his expressive communication.

Overcoming barriers by structuring the environment

Why use structure?

Increasing structure within the environment provides predictability and reduces confusion. It can promote independence, understanding and communication, and reduce anxiety. Often when we talk about structure and specifically 'structured teaching', it is in relation to the TEACCH® approach.

The TEACCH® approach

TEACCH® stands for 'Treatment and Education of Autistic and Communication – Handicapped Children', whilst the word 'handicapped' can feel jarring it is a helpful approach to consider when we are thinking about adapting the environment. A key element of the approach focusses on understanding the 'culture of autism'. This emphasises the unique strengths and needs of Autistic individuals and considers how the environment and everyday activities need to be adapted to meet these needs. The TEACCH® programme is based at the University of North Carolina and is used across the whole state of North Carolina for Autistic people across the lifespan (Mesibov and Shea, 2010). I have attended the TEACCH® training programme twice with Gary Mesibov and found the course truly inspirational. For more information about TEACCH® see www.teacch.com. The TEACCH® approach is used with Autistic people of all ages and stages from infants to adults. The approach is often used alongside other interventions (it is one tool in your toolbox). If you are familiar with special schools or specialist resource bases, often the environment is set up in a particular way with workstations for each student. Much of this draws upon the TEACCH® approach and key principles.

The TEACCH® approach has five key elements:

- **Physical structure** – This relates to the structure in place within the child or young person's actual environment; this could be the classroom or your home. We all benefit from physical structure in the environment to help us feel organised and understand what is happening, for example, a line on the train platform to show where we need to stand behind or a clear indication of what side to go up or down the stairs. The TEACCH® approach states that for Autistic people, physical structure gives meaning to the environment through increasing predictability; it makes the environment more organised. The use of structure can support a child or young person's understanding of what is expected in that environment.
- **Visual schedules or timetables** – Schedules, or as they are often known, visual timetables, are a visual representation of what is happening during the day, for example, the morning routine of nursery. Visual timetables can be pictures, written

or objects, according to the individual's level of symbolic understanding. Visual timetables aim to increase predictability, help a child understand when changes are going to happen, encourage independence and reduce anxiety.

- **Activity systems** – In our daily lives we all use lists of what we need to do as part of certain tasks. The TEACCH® approach states that Autistic people benefit from tasks being presented in a visual way to show what needs to be done and in what order; this is referred to as the activity or work system. As part of this, the student is shown how much work needs to be completed, the sequence the work needs to be carried out in and when the work is finished, and shows the child or young person what they need to do next.
- **Structured activities and tasks** – Within structured activities there is no need for verbal instruction as the visual structure provides a clear outline of the task so that the child is able to complete tasks independently without verbal prompting. The aim is to increase independence and participation.
- **Strengths and interests** – Incorporating an Autistic child's strengths and interests is a key part of the approach. There is an emphasis on using interests to help children engage in other activities; for example, using favourite characters as part of a schedule to increase motivation to engage with it.

The world can be a confusing place for Autistic children. Imagine yourself in a totally different country; perhaps everyone is speaking a different language, and you can't read the signs or understand what is happening. You don't understand the culture of the place you are in and are not sure where you are meant to be going and what you are meant to be doing. You feel lost and confused. Then you find yourself a map, start understanding a few key words and everything starts to make a bit more sense. Phew! You start to relax a little. Perhaps it is not so stressful after all. In the same way as you finding your map and understanding what was going on, we can add structure to make the environment easier to understand and more predictable. This means that children can do the following:

- Understand what we want them to do
- Have less anxiety – remember confusion can lead to anxiety
- Partake in daily activities
- Learn independence – we can use structure to help a child learn and carry out tasks independently although it is important to note that independence is not always the aim

Turn now to activity sheets (E:9)–(E:13; pages 80–89), which provide strategies and activities to increase the structure in your environment:

(E:9) – Structuring the learning environment – let's make a plan
(E:10) – Structuring the learning environment – top tips
(E:11) – Structuring a one-on-one area using a workstation
(E:12) – Structuring one-on-one activities
(E:13) – Supporting changes in the routine

Activity

Complete the planning sheet as part of (E:9).

Are there any other ways you can increase structure for the Autistic children you work with?

Use (E:15) to plan out implementation of any activities or strategies in the environment.

E:1 Environment activity sheet 1. Using objects to support understanding

E:1

Familiar objects can be used successfully with Autistic children as cues to help their understanding. This may be understanding of what is happening next, who is coming to see them, where they are going next, and so on. This can help reduce anxiety and increase predictability of the routine as well as help children learn to understand the world. Objects used to support understanding in this way are often referred to as 'objects of reference'. Adults working with an Autistic child using 'objects of reference' would typically have a bag of meaningful objects for the child that they would show to support understanding of the routine. Objects can represent people, activities, different times of the day and places but they need to be meaningful and personalised for the child.

How to use objects

- Start off by thinking of the routine of the day and which parts would be useful to have an object represent it, for example:
  - Nappy change/toilet time
  - Outside play
  - Snack/lunch
  - Parent
  - Music
- Talk to parents to see which objects you can overlap on. Consistency between home and school is key to supporting understanding.
- Think about the properties of the object as it can be helpful for there to be visual and tactile information as part of the object. For some children tactile information is more meaningful, and a piece of blanket stuck to a small board may be a useful way to signify naptime rather than a soft toy.
- When introducing objects, it is important to consider whether the item is meaningful and relevant for the child; for example, choosing a ball to represent outside play for a child who is not interested in balls will not signify 'outside' in a relevant way.

When to use objects

- Use objects before the activity is going to happen to support understanding. Show the object and say the word; for example, every time before snack, show a spoon and say 'snack time'.

How to step it up

If you feel that a child confidently understands objects, it may be worth introducing photos and pictures alongside these with the aim to transition to just photos or pictures. The ability to do this depends on a child's symbolic representation and how easily they understand that a picture, miniature or object relates to the activity. See the hierarchy of symbolic representation on page 56 of this chapter.

Materials needed

- Meaningful objects for the child
- Bag to store them

E:2 Environment activity sheet 2. Using photos to help understanding

E:2

Photos are used widely with Autistic children. As highlighted earlier in this chapter, Autistic children are visual learners, so this plays to their strengths. We talk about using photos and pictures across a range of activity sheets in this manual. As well as supporting understanding, pictures are also often used to help a child's expressive communication (more on this in Chapter 4). Ensure that a child has the symbolic understanding before choosing to use photographs and pictures. Remember that clear photos are easier to understand than abstract symbols. The photographs need to be meaningful to the child. If you are taking photos of familiar objects, make sure that they are not on a crowded or busy background.

How do photos help?

- Unlike a spoken word, which disappears, a picture provides a permanent representation and builds on the philosophy of '*show me, don't tell me*'.
- Using photographs and pictures may be implemented as part of a wider target of using a first/then board or a visual timetable – (E:3) and (E:5).
- In an environment that can feel overwhelming photographs can offer some predictability.

When to use photographs

- Photographs and pictures are helpful at any time during the day as part of the routine. They can be especially important at transition times or as part of a first/then board or visual timetable. It can be helpful to have photos of the nursery and key worker at home and a picture of home and the person picking them up at nursery.
- Sometimes when we first introduce photos or pictures, it can be helpful for staff to wear a lanyard with the symbols easily accessible on it so that they can be shown in the moment.

Tips

- As the child becomes accustomed to photographs, you could use them as part of a sequence first/then board or visual timetable.
- As children get older and particularly if they have an interest in letters, make sure that you have the written words alongside the photograph.
- Make sure that you say the word at the same time as the photograph, e.g. when you show a photo of lunch say 'lunchtime'.

Materials needed

- Camera and photographs
- Laminator

E:3 Environment activity sheet 3. Using a first/then board

E:3

A first/then board presents what we need to do now (first) and what we will do next (then) in a visual way. The board could be a laminated piece of card with attached pictures on or simply a whiteboard or piece of paper with the objects drawn or written on it. You can print the first/then board on page 68 (and see online support materials) to use in your setting.

What is a first/then board for?

The first/then board helps children understand the sequence of activities, for example, first story then bubbles. Introducing a first/then board can help with a number of areas including the following:

- Moving a child's attention between activities and understanding when things are finished – you can use the first/then board in conjunction with the strategies outlined on (E:4) around finishing activities
- Using the language first/then to help children with sequencing and understanding what's next
- Completing a less-preferred activity when there is a motivating activity next, for example, first wash hands then snack

How to use a first/then board

- Start off by using it with two activities that the child likes, for example, first bubbles then ball. I often see first/then not work when we don't use motivating activities.
- Keep your language simple: 'First bubbles then ball'.
- When the first activity is finished, use a one-minute warning and countdown – five, four, three, two, one – bubbles are finished (with gesture), remove the picture, then show the next one.
- Gradually extend to use the preferred activity second to encourage completion of the first activity.

When to use the board: You can use the first/then board throughout the day, but it can be especially helpful at transition times.

How to step it up

A first/then board (see Figure 3.2) can be a tool to help children move onto using a longer timetable or first/then/then as part of a structured activity. Sharing this strategy with parents can be extremely helpful if they don't already use one. Many parents I have worked with have fed back that using a finished countdown and first/then board has had a significant impact on the number of meltdowns their child has and makes situations like leaving the park much easier. Many children I meet ask 'what's next?' throughout the day; using a first/then board is a really helpful way to reduce the anxiety associated with this.

Materials needed

- First/then board (template for you to copy and use on the next page) and photos or symbols
- Whiteboard and pens as an alternative

First/then board

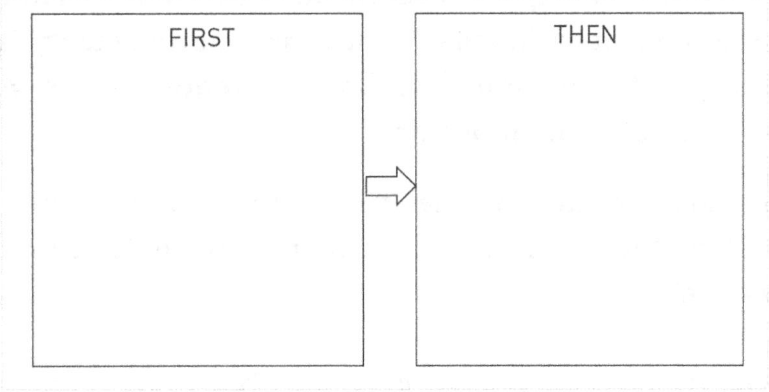

Figure 3.2

E:4 Environment activity sheet 4. Understanding the concept 'finished' and using a countdown

E:4

Transition times can be hard for Autistic children. Recognising that this is not a child being difficult or not listening is important. Monotropism plays a role in children becoming intensely absorbed in their interests and finding it hard to move on. Reducing anxiety around transition times is important in supporting Autistic children. Think of all the times in the day that an activity comes to an end and another one starts, all of these changes and separations from activities can be stressful. Whilst we can reduce unnecessary transitions in the day there will be times when understanding the concept of 'finished' is really important. This is important as many Autistic children find it difficult to know when something has finished, and it is time to move onto something new. A first/then board definitely helps with this, but it is also helpful to teach children the words and actions associated with the concept of 'finished'. Knowing that an activity is going to finish can reduce stress around transition times and also reduce stress when it is time to leave an object or setting and move on.

This relates to the 'show me and tell me' idea as often, when a child is busy playing and the adult is telling them it is time to finish, they haven't heard or engaged with the message at all.

How to help children understand the concept 'finished'

1. Get down to the child's level, say his or her name, and show your finger indicating one minute: *'Amy, one minute with cars'*. Repeat several times.
2. Still at their level say 'five, four, three, two, one (whilst showing your fingers, counting down), finished'. When you say 'finished', use a clear hand gesture. Say 'cars have finished' whilst placing the cars into a finished box or bag. Putting the objects in the box is important as they are then out of sight. Some children benefit from using a countdown timer (there are lots of apps that do this or you can use a sand timer).
3. Say it is time for blocks (and present next activity quickly). It is important that this is also something that they enjoy and is motivating to them.
   - **Be consistent** – It is extremely helpful if every member of staff can use a consistent routine (same words and actions) to communicate when an activity is finished. Consistency will help a child understand much quicker.

- **What's next** – It is important for the child to know what is happening next rather than finishing and having nothing to move onto. Often parents and educators say, '*Oh, he is really struggling to finish an activity*'. Think of yourself if you finish something you like doing; it is good to have something else to do. Similarly for the child, remember to show them what they can do next; for example, bubbles have finished, and it is time for books.

When to use 'finished'

- Use 'finished' at the end of the activity.
- Using a countdown for 'finished' will gradually become incorporated into your use of a first/then board and visual timetable. You will find that it is a useful tool to use in many situations.

Materials needed

- 'Finished' bag or box

E:5 Environment activity sheet 5. Using a visual timetable

E:5

A visual timetable is a structured way to represent the daily routine in a visual format. The use of a visual timetable can help increase predictability, and through this reduce uncertainty and anxiety. A visual timetable helps children understand what is happening next. Using a visual timetable plays to an Autistic child's visual strengths. Visual timetables are relevant for all Autistic children whatever their level of communication; we need to alter how we present the information to them. I have often heard people say that a particular child doesn't need a timetable, only later to wonder why they are struggling when it is time to finish or transition or when they are asking 'what's next?' throughout the day. Visual timetables don't have to be pictures. I worked with an Autistic 18-year-old doing her A-levels who was delighted to have created her own whiteboard timetable by the door of her room with a list that she would check off throughout the day.

A visual timetable can be made up of the following:

- Objects
- Photographs
- Symbols
- Words

It could be drawn on a whiteboard. It can be organised horizontally or vertically, and it can represent a whole day or a shorter section of time (see Figure 3.3).

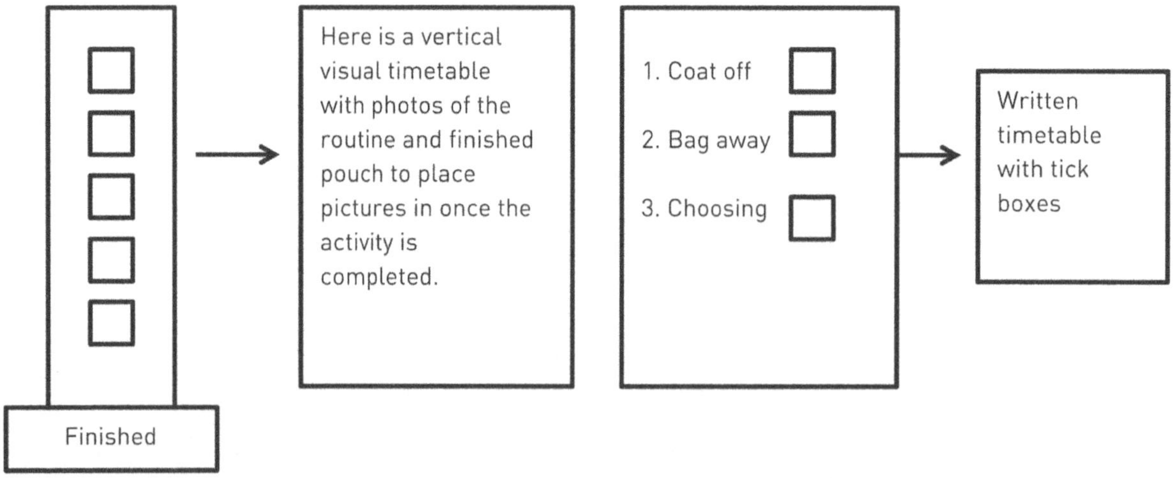

Figure 3.3

When setting up a visual timetable you need to consider the following:

- What is the child's level of symbolic understanding?
- How will you organise the pictures?
- Is it the timetable for the whole class or for a particular child? These are different and I would always recommend personalising a timetable for an individual child.
- How will the child interact with the timetable, for example, ticking off each activity, taking it off the picture strip and placing it in the 'finished' box? This part is important as if the timetable is on the wall and the pictures and symbols aren't removed it fails to show the passing of time and shifting between activities.

Materials needed

- Photos or symbols
- Whiteboard

E:6 Environment activity sheet 6. Understanding the concept of 'wait' and using a wait card

E:6

'Waiting' is a difficult concept to understand. In my experience it can be a barrier for Autistic children in daily activities where situations that require waiting can lead to distress. This can also have a big impact on parents' lives; when children are struggling to wait for a bus or in the shopping queue, this can also be stressful for the child. The tricky thing about waiting is that it is quite an abstract concept. You can't see 'wait' in the same way you can 'drink' or 'snack'. We need to be creative to think about how we can make the concept 'wait' more concrete.

We also need to make reasonable adjustments and ask ourselves if we can limit the times a child needs to wait.

When we think about waiting, we need to consider if a child knows what they are waiting for and how long they have to wait for. Is this information clear and available to them?

Teach 'waiting' at the right time

- Often, we are asking children to wait at a time when they are already finding it difficult, e.g. they are already not waiting, e.g. we are saying, 'Wait, wait', whilst they are trying to push their way in front of another child in the queue for the slide.
- We need to start commenting on when children are waiting in positive situations, for example, waiting for a snack or waiting at the traffic lights. Make comments like 'I am waiting for snack' and use gestures to support this.
- We can focus specifically on waiting in games and positive predictable activities.

Top tips

- Make it visual. Use a consistent gesture to accompany your words.
- Be clear with your communication, avoid language that is even more abstract, e.g. 'we are waiting, let's do that later'. 'Later' is even more abstract and confusing than 'wait'!
- Use a wait card. This is typically a card like the one that follows (with a red coloured background). Every time children are waiting, show them the card as a prompt. Use consistent language, for example, 'Waiting' or 'I am waiting'. Remember to tell a child what they are waiting for. It doesn't have to be a wait card, it could be an object that symbolises waiting for a child or an object that is comforting to hold.

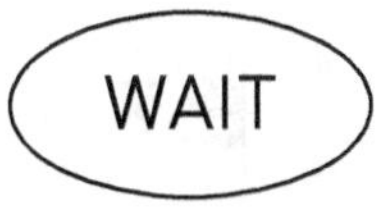

- How long am I waiting for? Sand timers and countdown timers also have the benefit of showing a child how long they need to wait.

- Consider how long you expect a child to wait. Be realistic; start with a short time and gradually increase it.
- Tell the children what is happening after they are waiting; this may be clear, but you could provide a visual reminder, for example, with a first/then board (E:3) or by using photographs to support understanding (E:4); for example, 'waiting for a snack'.
- Remember to say what is happening in the order that it is happening.
- Give specific praise rather than using phrases like 'good job'. This can be particularly helpful as it provides clear, concrete feedback about what a child has done well, reducing ambiguity and supporting understanding. When we highlight specific behaviours this helps children recognise their strengths and build confidence within a supportive and predictable environment.

Materials needed

- Wait card

E:7 Environment activity sheet 7. Using visuals to support taking part in everyday activities

E:7

We know that using visuals can help children with daily routines. Knowing what happens next can reduce anxiety and increase confidence along with a range of other skills. We can use visuals to support taking part in everyday activities; these work well in conjunction with the home setting. Visuals can support with executive functioning and planning, which becomes more important as children get older.

A timetable, as described in (E:5), can be used to break down everyday activities. Visuals are commonly used as part of the following everyday sequences:

- Toileting
- Getting dressed
- Leaving and getting to the nursery
- Bedtime routine
- Morning routine

Using a motivator at the end of the sequence is helpful to support children. For example:

- Breakfast
- Clothes on
- Clean teeth
- Shoes on
- Five minutes of TV

As with (E:5) this could be on a vertical or a horizontal timetable either in a fixed point or on a strip that can be moved around. Don't worry if you don't have the individual symbols or pictures to hand. Draw the routine out on the whiteboard.

Activity

Think of a child in your setting; how could visual supports help them participate in routines?

Working together on participation in daily routines is a good way to collaborate between home and nursery. Often these areas are targeted with support from an OT. Daily activities such as toileting or dressing (if the child is developmentally ready) can be great shared goals to target. The use of visual support can be helpful to show the child what the routine is and provide predictability and certainty as part of this.

Materials needed

- Photographs or symbols
- Whiteboard and pens

E:8 Environment activity sheet 8. Language for routines

E:8

Adding language to routines and activities can be a powerful strategy to help children develop and build understanding of language. Modelling consistent words and phrases at certain times of the day and in certain activities also provides children with a model of what they need to say and do. Routines are consistent, which then allows for regular opportunities for children to hear the same words, which allows for language learning.

One of the most powerful, easy-to-use strategies to support a child's understanding is to reduce your language when you are talking. Often, we don't realise that we are using long sentences, which makes it hard for a child to understand or latch onto the particular word as part of the routine. For example, at a transition time saying, 'Come on Sam you need to finish that up we need to go and get a snack', you could instead get down to Sam's level and say 'Snack' (whilst showing the picture.

Language is not just talking

Adding gestures and pointing is another visual way of helping a child understand the words and environment.

Top tips for adding language to routines

- Use less language.
- Repeat key words and phrases.
- Talk about what a child is doing – this helps children learn action words and match language to their activity
- Model language that is useful to a child, e.g. if they are stuck say 'help'. Model language from the child's perspective (declarative language). More on this in Chapter 4.
- Add gestures.
- Be consistent in the language you use.
- Be musical and creative, for example, singing a tidy-up song or hello or good-bye song every day. Routine songs can help a child understand the routine.
- Use the child's interests; add language to routines that are motivating to them.

Remember to match your use of language to the child's level of language. This will help you best support their understanding. For example, for a child who is at an early stage of communication, instead of saying 'let's go and wash hands now; our hands are all dirty', try pointing at the dirty hands, saying 'dirty', then pointing to the sink and saying 'let's wash hands' (whilst using a gesture and using a visual support). To begin with it can feel quite unnatural to be saying less; think of it as communicating at the right level for the child.

Materials needed

- None

E:9 Environment activity sheet 9. Structuring the learning environment – let's make a plan

E:9

Earlier in the chapter we discussed the TEACCH® approach and one of the key principles of structuring the environment. Within the TEACCH® approach this is referred to as the 'physical structure' and refers to the actual surroundings and arrangement of an Autistic person's learning or home environment. We can structure the environment to include different areas for work, snack, play, calming area, books or whichever areas that are specific to your environment.

We know that structure can help to accomplish the following:

- Reduce anxiety
- Increase understanding
- Promote participation

Planning the environment

Learning environments often have quite clear boundaries in terms of different areas, for example, home corner, snack area, toilet and hand washing. These clearly defined 'zoned' areas can be helpful for Autistic children.

The aim in planning the environment is to think about whether we can make any of the areas any clearer in terms of their function. One of the areas that I often see as a barrier is when children have to wait, and it is not clear where and how long for. A simple bit of tape on the floor can really make the environment a bit clearer.

Turn to the planning sheet on page 81, which can be photocopied.

- Draw out your learning space.
- Label the different areas.
- From your plan is it clear what each area is for?
- What areas already have a clear structure, and what areas could be clearer? Use the planning sheet to think about your space.
- Is there any furniture you could use to create clearer 'zones' (e.g. instead of having a bookcase against the wall, turn it to create a clearer reading corner)?
- Think about how you can label the areas using visual supports.

Activity

Draw your space, clearly label different areas and think about how you can add structure to the environment.

E:10 Environment activity sheet 10. Structuring the learning environment – top tips

E:10

We know that adding structure to the learning environment is a positive strategy for Autistic children. This is a key feature of the TEACCH® approach.

Now that you have completed your plan (E:8), think about which areas in your learning environment you can bring more structure to.

Activity

Brainstorm how you can bring more structure to your environment.
Add your ideas to (E:9). The ideas that follow may be relevant to your setting.

Boundaries

It may feel that the areas of the classroom are clearly defined; think about it from the perspective of an Autistic child. Would it make sense? Could you add any physical markers, for example, masking tape on the floor, or position the furniture in a certain way so that each area is clearly defined?

Lining up

Using tape on the floor to make a line to show children where to stand can be a helpful and simple way to add structure to the environment. You could also use a visual support to indicate who is going to go first in the line and also a wait card (E:6).

Circle time

Using a carpet spot or square, cushion or even a sticker on the floor can be a helpful way to show a child where he or she needs to sit.

Colours

Using different-colour tables and chairs, or even adding a different colour tablecloth, can be a helpful way of creating different 'zones' in the environment. This can also help a child understand different activities in the same space; for example, a yellow table covering could indicate snack, and blue could indicate messy play.

Quiet area

Having a clearly defined quiet 'low arousal' area can be helpful for Autistic children within the nursery as this can help children to feel more in control and less overwhelmed. When I do nursery observations and visits, I always see the benefit of having a quiet zone as this can build in opportunities for breaks for a child to recharge. It is important that access to this area is freely available and should not be something that a child needs to earn or have as a reward. This area could have beanbags or a tent. Within this quiet area, consider the amount of information on display. It may be that you choose neutral colours without decoration on the walls within this area so that it is less visually stimulating. Years ago, I worked in a special school for Autistic children where they consistently used the Low Arousal Approach as part of their curriculum. All the classroom walls were blue and there were minimal visual distractions, particularly in the quiet or calm area; it made a real difference.

Outside play

Outside play naturally lends itself to having clearly defined different areas: for example, messy sand and water, a pretend play area with a toy house and physical play. If you have bikes or equipment that requires children to take turns, consider using a timer or turn-taking board (Chapter 5; S:8) to create predictability around this.

Materials needed

- Based on your planning outlined in (E:9)

E:11 Environment activity sheet 11. Structuring a one-on-one area using a workstation

E:11

A workstation is a key part of the structured teaching method outlined as part of the TEACCH® approach. Like much of the TEACCH® philosophy, using a workstation incorporates routine, visual cues, routine and structure as well as limiting distractions. Use of a workstation aims to help Autistic children to partake in learning by supporting independent, focussed and organised learning. The goal of this is not solely independence but to create a structured and reduced distraction area to support children in accessing learning. If your local area has an Autism outreach service, this may be something that a teacher is able to support you with. This activity sheet provides a brief overview.

The workstation shows a child these steps:

- What I need to do
- How much work there is to do
- How I know that I have finished
- What happens next

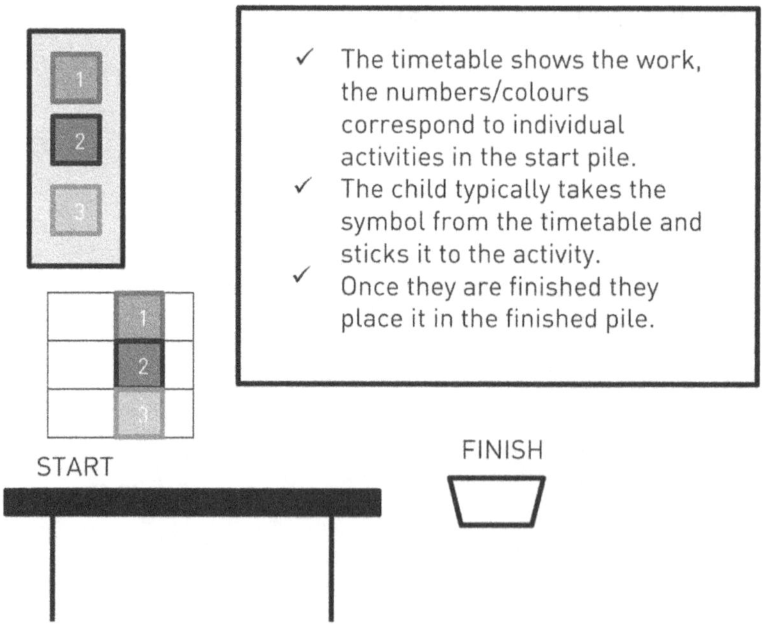

Figure 3.4 Example of a workstation

Providing this clear structure helps to reduce anxiety and support a child's ability to complete tasks. In my experience workstations are often used incorrectly and this can be really unhelpful. Instead of focussing on activities that children can complete independently, they become one-on-one teaching areas or a storage area for toys and activities. A workstation should focus on activities a child can complete on their own, e.g. a favourite puzzle or activity working left to right.

What activities to use

- Use activities that a child is interested in, so they are able to carry them out with minimal support. This can help children to feel the satisfaction of completion.
- Puzzles and manipulation tasks work well.
- Shoebox tasks, available to purchase, can also work well.
- Any activity can be adapted to be a workstation activity.

Materials needed

- Table
- Plastic trays
- Plastic wallets for activities

E:12 Environment activity sheet 12. Structuring one-on-one activities

E:12

We can use structure and visual support to encourage a child to take part within an activity. This is particularly helpful for children who benefit from seeing what is coming next. By stepping back and having clear steps of what is coming a child is able to have the intrinsic satisfaction of completing the task without needing to be prompted all the way.

Sometimes visuals like this are called a task planner; essentially this is like a visual timetable for within the activity. It breaks the activity down to show the child each component part. This is easily adapted to many activities and can be used in conjunction with other children as part of a small group. Figure 3.5 is an example of a hand-drawn out visual structuring the activity of a lemonade volcano. You can also use a task planner which can be printed out.

Materials needed

- Whiteboard
- Whiteboard pens
- Task planner template

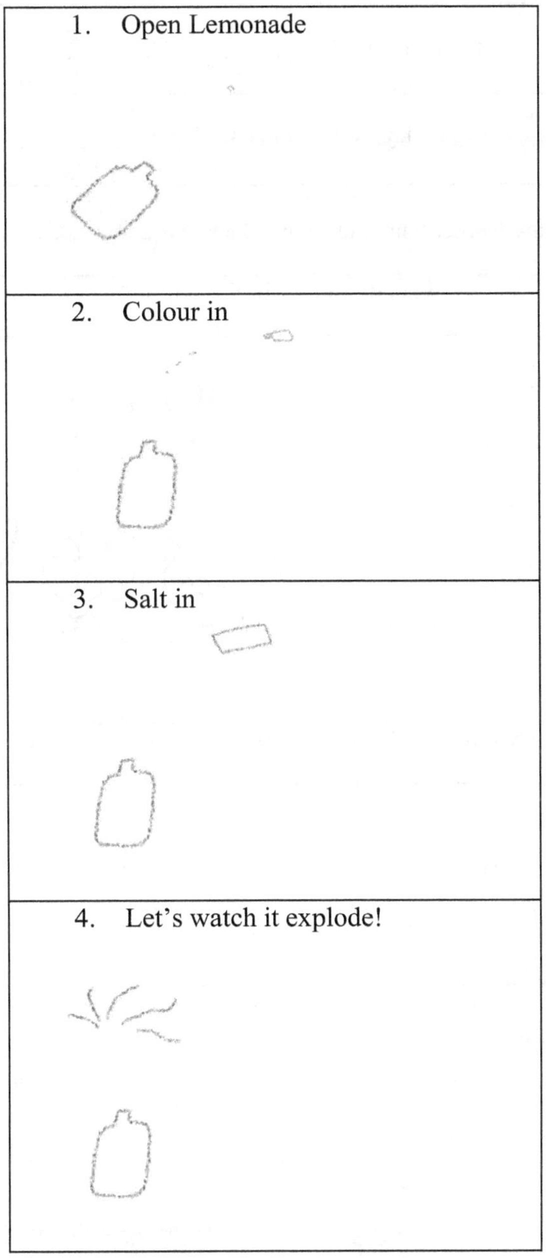

Figure 3.5 Hand-drawn visual of making a lemonade volcano

What activity are we doing? ......Making fruit salad ....

Where are we doing the activity? ......In the outdoor kitchen ....

Who will be there? ......My key worker Sam and friends Jack and Leo.........

What do I need for the activity?

1. ....Bowl..........................
2. ....Knife..........................
3. .... Apple........................
4. ....Banana..........................
5. ....Orange........................
6. ....Grapes........................

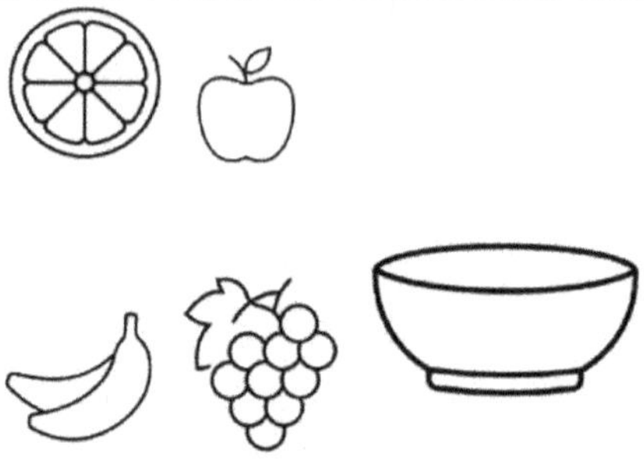

What do I need to do? What are the steps involved?

Step 1 ....Get Bowl ....

Step 2 ....Peel and cut fruit ....

Step 3 ....Put it in the bowl and mix it ....

Step 4 ....Eat it with my friends, YUM YUM..........................

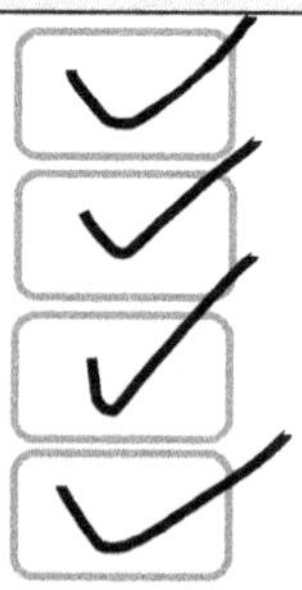

How long for:

5 minutes
We can watch the sand timer

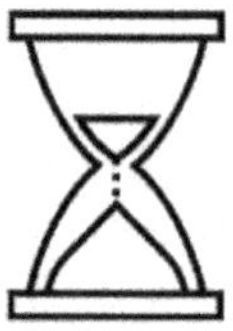

What's next:

Wash hands and then free choice

Figure 3.6 Sample task planner completed for making a fruit salad

E:13 Environment activity sheet 13. Supporting changes in the routine

E:13

By supporting routines and building in consistency and predictability we are able to reduce anxiety. However, sometimes there are unexpected changes to the routine, for example, a trip out with the nursery or a change to the usual activities such as a Christmas activity or a new teacher or a teacher going on maternity leave. Given how important certainty is for Autistic children, it is important that as educators we have tools to help prepare children for changes to the routine.

Having good communication with parents is a key first step as it is vital to let parents know any upcoming changes so that these can be supported rather than being suddenly sprung upon a child. Remember that even small changes can have a big impact on a child so working out a good way to communicate what is happening is important.

We can support children's understanding of changes by using the following strategies:

- Use visual supports to help prepare a child. For example, for a trip have an individual timetable of the day's routine including mode of transpiration, activities and what is happening at the end. Take a whiteboard as backup to be able to draw out what is happening as needed. Many places such as museums or tourist attractions have a ready-made social story on their website which is really helpful. It is always worth contacting them to check.
- If it is a school trip, parents could visit with the child before. I worked once with a child who started doing this for the first few visits. His family visited the place (a museum in Central London) at the weekend and took a series of photos, which were then printed out and added to a social story to support him (Gray, 2019). This prepared the child effectively and significantly reduced anxiety before the trip.
- You can prepare children for new experiences using social stories (Gray, 2019). More on social stories in E:14.
- Using a calendar or schedule for the week can also be helpful in helping a child understand changes to the routine. For example, if Mum has to go away, being able to show visually what days she will be at home and then who will be at home on the other days is helpful. This could be linked to a social story of what happens when Mum is away. Similarly using the calendar to show when it is Christmas or Halloween will be helpful.

E:14 Environment activity sheet 14. Using social stories

E:14

(Gray, 2019)

Social stories were originally developed by Carol Gray in 1991. They are a very helpful tool to support understanding and reduce anxiety in Autistic children. Social stories help to make sense of confusing situations, reduce anxiety around change and uncertainty and build understanding over time. A social story is always personalised and for nursery aged children should include pictures. They can be helpful to support a child in understanding a new situation or making sense of a social situation. For example, going on holiday, going to the dentist, what happens with the fire alarm, going on a school trip or even starting at a new school. They are written in a concrete and person-first way at the right language level to support an individual child and reduce anxiety.

Unfortunately, social stories can be misused at times and often I have seen really poor examples that dictate behaviour, so instead of gently describing a social situation the story becomes a list of demands. Or the story will be written in a way so as to force compliance. Or sometimes instead of using first-person language they use 'you'. Often, I see generic social stories downloaded from the internet that don't work for a child because they are not personalised, or they are far too complex. It is really important that if you are going to write a social story you read more about how to do it, and it is done in a way that is not harmful. They should be thought of as a 'map' to support and enable a child to navigate, not a list of demands or script that demands compliance.

Key elements of social stories:

Purpose: The social story will explain what will happen, who is involved, where it occurs and why. It might also explain what different people might be thinking and feeling.

Key components: The social story should outline perspectives (at the right language and developmental level) and provide positive, non-judgemental guidance as opposed to rules.

Structure: The social story needs to be written in a simple format, with pictures to make events more predictable. It does not need to be too long.

Use: They are effective in helping a child prepare for change, navigate social situations or build on skills. They are not a list of rules.

Social stories include several core elements including:

- Descriptive sentences that state facts about a situation; these are written in a clear and unambiguous way
- Perspective sentences that add information about the thoughts, feelings and reactions of others
- Coaching sentences that gently guide the reader to a positive response

Top tips for writing social stories:

- Write from the child's perspective at the right language level or from a neutral third-person's perspective. Avoid 'you'.
- Help the child with the 'why' by providing information about the social context to support a child's understanding.
- Read before the situation not at times of stress.
- Use descriptive and reassuring language, focus on describing not directing language.
- Keep it short and simple, one concept per story.
- Do not tell a child what they should/shouldn't do in a directive way.
- Tailor the story to a child's interests, make it personal and age appropriate.
- Focus on understanding and not performance.
- Read the story frequently and help the child to be involved, e.g. drawing a picture or selecting pictures for it.

E:15 Environment activity sheet 15. Strategy sheet template

E:15

Child's name:
Aim: (The aim for the child) Rationale: (Why this is important) Strategy/activity to be introduced: How this will help: What will be different: (For the child) How to implement: (Clear steps and how to share)

Chapter 3 summary

- The education environment and early years curriculum can be stressful and overwhelming for Autistic children. We need to make reasonable adjustments to reduce barriers and enable participation.
- We can make positive changes to the environment to make it more predictable for Autistic children.
- We can use an Autistic child's strength in visual processing and introduce a range of visual supports depending on their level of symbolic representation.
- Visual supports don't need to be complicated; they could just be a whiteboard and pen.
- Increasing structure as part of the routine helps increase the child's understanding of the environment.
- Activity sheets (E:1)–(E:14) all provide practical tips on how to support understanding and make the learning environment more accessible for Autistic children.

References

Beardon, L. 2017. *Autism and Asperger Syndrome in Adults.* 2nd ed. Sheffield: Sheldon Press.

Gray, C. 2019. *Carol Gray Social Stories*. https://carolgraysocialstories.com/.

Mesibov, G.B. and Shea, V. 2010. The TEACCH® program in the era of evidence-based practice. *Journal of Autism and Developmental Disorders*, *40*(5), pp.570–579.

4

Communication skills

Chapter 4 provides the following:

- An overview of how communication develops
- Early communication skills
- Different styles of language learning: Gestalt Language Processing
- Introducing Alternative and Augmentative Communication
- Practical case studies to illustrate strengths and differences in communication profiles of Autistic children
- Activity sheets:
  (C:1) – Developing joint and shared attention
  (C:2) – The power of pausing
  (C:3) – Imitation 'copy me'!
  (C:4) – Making chances to communicate – offering choices
  (C:5) – Making chances to communicate – giving
  (C:6) – Making chances to communicate – a bit at a time
  (C:7) – Ready, steady, go games
  (C:8) – Stop/go games
  (C:9) – Making choices with a choosing board
  (C:10) – Asking for help
  (C:11) – Using songs
  (C:12) – Adding language
  (C:13) – Using action words
  (C:14) – Supporting gestalt language processors
  (C:15) – Let's create
  (C:16) – Using an about-me book or 'chat book'

DOI: 10.4324/9781003627760-4

Development of communication

Communication develops even before a child is born; in the womb babies are becoming familiar with the native language spoken in their environment. From soon after birth babies develop their sociocognitive skills, then comes receptive language (understanding) and typically around 12 months expressive language (spoken language when first words appear). Typically, children start to understand words before they are able to say them. Long before children are talking, they are developing important skills that are foundations of communication. Receptive and expressive language are self-explanatory, but what do we mean by sociocognitive skills?

Sociocognitive skills relate to early emerging skills in engaging and interacting with others; they are important skills in the development of communication, social interaction and play. In neurotypical children these skills are innate and are crucial to the development of both language and social communication. These skills include (amongst others) joint and shared attention and social responsiveness in addition to gesture and symbolic understanding. These skills all play a part in two-way communication. Typically, children do not need to learn these skills; they just develop them. Think of a baby or young child of one year old; typically, when you smile at them, they smile at you, or if you look or point to an item out of sight, they are intrigued and interested to know what you are looking at. Neurotypical children are naturally wired to be social, and from an early age, long before they can talk, are learning how to use these skills.

We know that communication is so much more than words. Gestures, symbolic understanding and joint and shared attention all play a huge part in the development of typical communication. As an SLT, I am often asked about what sounds a child should be saying and questions relating to the mechanics of talking. Whilst SLTs do have a role in this, so much more of my work is around the building blocks of communication that happen a long time before we start to focus on how a word is pronounced and sounds.

Joint attention

Joint attention relates to the ability to share a focus of attention with someone else. In simple terms joint attention happens when two people focus on the same thing and both know about it. In practical terms a parent and young child may play together with a pop-up toy. The child looks at the toy, then looks towards the parent, and the parent responds by looking at the toy and the child. This back-and-forth sharing of attention allows both people to recognise that they are focused on the same thing.

Typically, joint attention emerges in young children towards the end of their first year of life and involves both responding to joint attention and initiating joint attention. These skills are important for developing attention and communication in a typical way and support looking and listening to activities together, learning new words and engaging in interaction with others. SLTs often talk about joint attention as a key part of communication and social interaction development. Whilst these are important skills it is important to acknowledge that in Autistic children joint attention can be different, it can develop at a later stage or develop in a different way. This does not mean that it is 'wrong' or not there, just that it is different.

In neurotypical children examples of joint attention might include things like a child pointing to something exciting like an aeroplane and looking back at the adult to share it with them. Or looking where someone else points or bringing a toy to show someone and looking from the toy to the adult and back. Do you remember in the first parent story in Chapter 2 where the mother talks about noticing differences in how her child shared attention and enjoyment with her:

> *My instinct was telling me that he was not sharing his enjoyment with me in the way that I saw other children do with their parents. For example, he would look up at an aeroplane in the sky and stay fixed on it until it disappeared. I would see other children look at that same aeroplane and then look back at their parent as though they were telling their parent 'look mummy/daddy, I see an aeroplane'.*

In my work with younger children I have noticed that joint attention in Autistic children can look different in a number of ways:

- Autistic children may share attention without eye contact; they may be close to you and communicate this in a different way. You can still be focussing on and sharing joy in the same object.
- They may show joint attention by bringing you objects that they are interested in, which also may not be accompanied with eye contact.
- They may share interests in other ways, and these may involve other forms of communication, e.g. not always typical gestures like pointing.
- Autistic children may have an intense shared interest in something that is motivating to them, not something that has been selected by the adult.

With this in mind it is important to tune into an Autistic child's interests and how they share joint attention with you. Joint attention supports the development of communication and interaction, relationship building and learning through social experiences. It is, however, really important not to force joint attention as that can increase anxiety, reduce trust and encourage masking. Recognising that it may look different and adapting your communication is key. See (C:1) for ideas of how to support joint attention in Autistic children.

Attention and listening versus joint attention

Joint attention is quite an abstract concept and isn't always something I often see educators attempting to develop. Sometimes there can be confusion between attention and listening skills and joint attention and it is important to clarify the difference. These skills are both relevant to communication so I will provide some clarity!

Often when I visit nurseries, staff have concerns that a child 'won't pay attention' or 'won't sit at a table or group time'. Naturally there is a tendency to want to develop attention and listening skills as they have such a big impact on other areas of development and this then becomes a goal as part of an individual education plan; for example, 'Jack will sit for ten minutes'. In many cases a goal like this is asking too much and is just not realistic. It also fails to take into account important factors like what Jack will be doing when he is sitting. Is he interested and motivated by this? Is it meaningful for him? As part of the typical school day children do need to develop their ability to pay attention to others as part of activities. However, it is important we go at the pace of the child and have realistic expectations.

Often sitting in a circle and listening to a story is not motivating or in line with a child's attention skills. Table 4.1 outlines stages of attention adapted from Cooper et al. (1978) and provides some simple strategies for each level. Whilst this is quite an old framework it remains relevant in terms of helping us to consider where a child is and what we are asking them to do in terms of their attention. If these don't match up a child will find it difficult to engage; quite simply, if the activity is not at the right level for their attention, we are not setting them up for success. Often the activities that we expect an Autistic child to engage in within an early years education environment are at a higher level (Level 5–Level 6) than their skills are at (Level 1–Level 4). This is not the case that a child is 'behind' and needs to 'work harder', it is just a reflection of differences in attention. It highlights the perspective that we need to be adapting the activity for the child.

Activity

Look at the stages of attention in Table 4.1. Think about a child you work with and think what level of attention they are at. Think about the activities they can and can't engage with. What is the difference?

In Chapter 1 we talked about monotropism and what this means for attention in Autistic children; it's important to keep this in mind. Monotropism (the narrow torch beam style of attention) means an Autistic child might focus very intently on one thing at a time that is highly motivating to them. In the nursery environment this shows up as intense interests and having a difficult time switching activities which can cause distress during transition times. We need to think about our expectations for activities and attention to ensure that Autistic children have opportunities to engage that are meaningful for them.

Table 4.1 Stages of attention, implications and support strategies (adapted from Cooper et al., 1978)

Stage of attention	*What this looks like*	*What the impact is*	*Support strategies*
Level 1 – Very distractible with fleeting attention only.	The child's attention is on whatever is their current interest and will be quickly shifted to anything new.	Unable to attend to any adult led tasks.	Find out what is interesting to the child. Follow his or her lead and incorporate these into what you are doing. See (C:1) and (C:2).
Level 2 – Attends to own choice of activity for a longer period of time but cuts self off from everything else.	Can concentrate on a task of their own choosing. A child at this stage does not have the ability to focus on more than one task. It is difficult for an adult to direct the child onto tasks that are not motivating for him or her.	Unable to engage with activities that are not interesting to them. Difficulties with transitions.	Before giving an instruction get down to the child's level and say his or her name. A visual prompt or touching his or her arm will also be a helpful cue. Use a countdown and strategies to support understanding around 'finished' (E:4).
Level 3 – Still single-channelled attention but begins to attend to adults.	Children at this stage will still focus on self-chosen activities, often for long periods, but they are starting to be able to shift their attention between activities with adult support.	Without adult support, will focus only on self-selected activities. Difficulties with transitions.	Gain the child's attention before giving any instructions or expecting a response. Call his or her name before speaking. Use a child's interests to encourage participation. Use a first/then board (E:3) and consistent use of countdown (E:4) to support understanding of the concept 'finished'.

Table 4.1 (Continued)

Stage of attention	*What this looks like*	*What the impact is*	*Support strategies*
Level 4 – Still single-channelled but able to shift attention between tasks with prompts.	Children at this stage begin to be able to control their own focus of attention. They require less adult support to shift their attention to and from activities.	Difficulties in attending flexibly to tasks.	Use visual prompts, e.g. a visual timetable (E:5) and photographs to support understanding (E:2). Give information in a clear sequence. Talk about things happening in the order that they occur.
Level 5 – Integrated attention for short periods of time.	Children at this stage have 'dual-channelled attention'; this means that they can be doing something whilst listening to an adult giving instructions. Able to cope with group situations.	Attention can still be quite short at times.	Encourage active listening; give specific praise for good listening.
Level 6 – Integrated attention well established.	A child at this stage has flexible attention and is able to sustain focus for lengthy periods of time. The child can integrate visual and auditory information with ease.	The child is able to focus in a way that allows them to engage with classroom learning in the way most children are expected to.	Encourage active questioning and processing of information.

We can support attention in Autistic children by:

- Understanding the role of monotropism and having strong interests
- Being realistic in our expectations when we think about what stage a child is at and match the activity. So, for a child with self-directed attention at Level 1 it is totally unrealistic to expect them to sit at circle time for a story. We need to be joining them in their interests.
- Remembering the goal is not just 'paying attention', ask yourself, 'what is the activity? Is it motivating? Is it meaningful?'
- Having predictable routines
- Supporting transitions
- Reducing demands when a child's attention is occupied

Development of communication in Autistic children

Autistic children develop communication differently than neurotypical children. Historically this has sometimes been viewed from a deficits perspective with negative language around 'disordered profiles' highlighting what Autistic children can't do rather than a strengths-based perspective of what they can. One of the key reasons for the updated second edition of this manual was to shift away from these outdated perspectives and provide insights into communication that are aligned with current thinking around Autism and Autistic communication styles.

Communication in Autistic children might look different than how it develops in other children. From the parent stories in Chapter 2 it is clear that milestones matter less and stepping away from these can be really helpful. Trying to measure a child's progress against norms that were not designed for them is likely to leave everyone feeling disheartened. Instead of comparing an Autistic child to milestones it can be helpful to gather information about areas of strength and difference. Using (I:1) and (I:2) we are able to consider a child's individual profile in terms of what's going well and what might feel harder.

We will think now about different features we see in the communication styles of Autistic children starting with Gestalt Language Processing.

Gestalt Language Processing

Gestalt Language Processing (GLP) is a framework around language learning that originated in linguistics and psychology. It is not an intervention programme or theory but has key principles that are important to be aware of as an early years educator. The work of Dr. Ann Peters, Barry Prizant and Marg Blanc has all been instrumental. In recent years it has become increasingly popular with parents and clinicians looking for strategies to support Autistic children who learn language through echolalia. I have found the GLP framework and associated strategies incredibly helpful in understanding and supporting Autistic children and have had real success in supporting children's language development with them.

Whilst GLP is generally viewed as very positive amongst SLTs who use it with Autistic children, a 2024 systematic review found no published research studies on its effectiveness; in simple terms this means that the key concepts come from descriptions rather than work reported in mainstream academic journals. This means that whilst there is a lot of anecdotal evidence to support GLP, the research evidence is still growing. The Royal College of Speech and Language Therapists describes GLP as a descriptive way of understanding some children's language use rather than a formal diagnosis or evidence-based intervention and suggests focussing on detailed communication profiles rather than labelling a child as a 'GLP'.

Let's turn now in more detail to look at what GLP is and think about why it is important for you to know about.

Development and stages

There are two main ways that children develop language. There is Analytic Language Processing (ALP) which is what is seen in neurotypical children where children learn words one at a time before building those words into phrases and then longer and longer sentences. The other way that some children develop language is through Gestalt Language Processing. Instead of learning one word at a time, gestalt language processors start communicating using chunks of language or 'gestalts'. In GLP, echolalia is an integral part of language development. The framework highlights that if children are developing language in a different way, they will need different strategies and supports. It is therefore important that if you are working with Autistic children, you are aware of this and have some understanding and strategies to provide support.

Gestalts are often phrases or songs copied from cartoons, books or YouTube clips, or language heard from family members or at nursery. A gestalt can be as short as a single word or as long as an entire story, but it is always processed as one unit of meaning that cannot be broken down into smaller parts. If a child is processing language in this way, you may not always understand what they are saying. Their language may sound like 'jargon' or babbling with lots of rich intonation. This is because gestalt language processors may tune in to the intonation, melody and rhythm of language more than the individual words. Sometimes GLP language processors may seem to use language that is out of context. This is because children pick up gestalts when they are linked to specific experiences or emotions, so cannot always be taken literally. As children progress through the stages of GLP, they gradually begin to break their gestalts down into smaller parts, which can then be recombined to create original, flexible language used as part of natural, spontaneous communication.

GLP is a normal and natural way to develop language. It is more common in Autistic children, but not all gestalt language processors are Autistic. Some gestalt language processors will move through the stages without needing support, whilst others will need additional support to move from one stage to the next. The framework outlines different stages that children move through whilst developing their language. The stages are predictable and eventually lead to flexible and spontaneous language. Table 4.2 summarises the stages of ALP and GLP language development.

Table 4.2 Stages of ALP and GLP language development (adapted from Blanc (2012, 2014) and informed by Prizant's work on echolalia and communicative development (Prizant, 1983; Prizant & Duchan, 1981)

Analytic Language Development	*Gestalt Language Development*
The basic unit of language is words: 1. Use of single words, e.g. 'ball' 2. Use of two-word combinations, e.g. 'mummy ball' 3. Use of emerging grammar in phrases, e.g. 'mummy give ball' 4. Use of first sentences, e.g. 'mummy give me the ball' 5. Use of more complex sentences/grammar, e.g. 'mummy gave me the ball'	The basic unit of language is 'chunks': 1. Use of echolalia to communicate 2. Breaking apart gestalts 3. Isolating single words and using single words and novel two-word combinations 4. Use of pre-sentence grammar in novel phrases 5. Use of advanced grammar in self-generated sentences 6. Use of more complex sentences/grammar

Sophia has a GLP language learning style, she loves Cocomelon nursery rhymes and singing. Table 4.3 highlights how she has moved through stages.

Table 4.3 Example of a GLP language learner at different stages

	Example: Sophia moving through stages 1–6
Stage 1: Whole gestalts	Sophia sings 'wheels on the bus go round and round' very loudly and tunefully. She is using this as a whole gestalt and tends to sing when excited or when she wants something.
Stage 2: Mitigations (which combines shortening, dividing and recombining)	Sophia starts saying 'wheels on the bus' or 'round and round'. She is often pausing and not using this as a whole gestalt.
Stage 3: Single words	Chunks are broken down into single words and Sophia is starting to make spontaneous two-word combinations, for example, 'red bus' and 'round'.
Stage 4: Original phrases	Sophia's phrases are now more flexible, but the grammar is not consistent, e.g. '*I want bus*', '*The bus is driving*'.
Stage 5: Original sentences	Sophia is starting to use more complex sentences, e.g. '*Let's put the people upstairs*', '*The red bus is going fast*'.
Stage 6. Complete grammar	Advanced language integration, e.g. '*I remember playing the wheels on the bus!*'

Tip

If you want to read in more detail about GLP, the Meaningful speech website (www.meaningfulspeech.com) is a helpful starting point and has many online courses and materials to access.

Signs that a child may have a GLP language learning style

You can look for signs about a child's language learning style. Observing and tuning into them are helpful first steps; have a pen and paper handy to jot down the language they use in different situations and interactions. A child may:

- Use words or phrases that sound copied (echolalia)
- Use the same phrases or parts of phrases
- Use out of context phrases
- Use unintelligible but tuneful strings of sound
- Use a melodic intonation pattern (can sound like singing)
- Sing or hum tunes (the words may not all be clear)
- Be very musical and enjoy singing and dancing
- May refer to themselves as 'you', e.g. they might say 'do you want a drink?' when they want a drink
- Sometimes seem to get stuck on certain single words
- Enjoy portions of songs or videos

Some children may be 'mixed' gestalt and analytic language processors which means they fall along a continuum between analytic language development and gestalt language development. They may use some language flexibly (i.e. word-by-word) whilst other language may be processed in chunks.

It is really important to recognise that children with a GLP language learning style are not just copying. The phrases they are using are used to communicate feeling, ask for help, cope with transitions and ultimately to stay safe and regulated.

Yafet is four years old. He is Autistic and has a GLP language learning style. Staff feel that he has made a lot of progress with his language skills and is able to communicate in sentences. Sometimes they aren't sure what he is trying to tell them as they realise that a lot of language is echoed from his favourite Julia Donaldson books. Yafet also echoes words that he has heard from his favourite television programmes and also the routine at nursery, for example, 'Good job, Yafet'. Now that staff realise that Yafet has a different language learning style, they are able to use strategies in play with him.

I remember working with a little boy many years ago who used the gestalt 'bangandthedirtisgone' (from the Cillit Bang advert). He tended to do this whilst tapping an adult's leg and it meant that he wanted to leave. When his mum said 'ok – you want to go! Let's go' he responded to her with smiling. Her response in terms of acknowledging and understanding his communication showed him that he had been understood.

Another example was a little girl who would say 'To infinity and beyond!' when very happy in her play. When adults responded with 'wow, you are excited let's play', or something similar, it showed her that she had been understood and that her communication partners were happy to join in.

All forms of communication are valid; some children learn language in chunks, and some learn language through building up single words. Our job is to understand the meaning of what a child is trying to convey and support their communication. We do not have to stop them using chunks of language. This is very important.

See (C:14) for tips on supporting children with a GLP style of language development.

Features of communication in Autistic children

We know that communication in Autistic children is different. That doesn't make it wrong or something that needs fixing. It is important that we have an awareness of differences so that we can tune into the children we work with. Through tuning in we can support children to communicate in a way that is meaningful to them whilst removing barriers around not being able to understand or communicate. Recognising difference also means that we can write targets in a way that is affirmative and aligns with Autistic communication.

We might see the following patterns in Autistic children:

- **Learning language through echolalia** (which we have already covered).
- **Finding it hard to 'ask for things'**: When children are non-speaking it can be hard for them to 'ask for things' to make their needs known. This can result in frustration and a child not being heard. I often meet children who may be very resourceful in trying to get their needs met, e.g. climbing to get the object they would like. A non-speaking child may reach to an object, take your hand or just stand near something they want but find it difficult to communicate another way. By tuning into their likes

and dislikes we can help them with communicating their preferences. Even when children have language, they may still struggle to 'ask' for things.

Salma is four and a half. She is Autistic and in her diagnostic report it says 'good language skills'. Although she has a detailed vocabulary, especially in relation to animals, which is one of her favourite topics, she finds it difficult to make requests. When she wants a drink, she will often ask an adult, 'Would you like a drink?' When stuck she will never ask for help. Recently her key worker noticed her doing a craft activity. When other children had the glue, she did not ask to have a turn and waited until it came near enough for her to reach over and take it.

- **Difficulties with processing and understanding language**: Autistic children may find it hard to understand language at times. Lots of language can also be really overwhelming. You might see:
  - Difficulties in following instructions (particularly those that are longer and more complex)
  - Difficulties in understanding non-literal language or language that is abstract. Whilst we don't tend to talk in idioms English is very abstract, and we don't always say what we mean and mean what we say. Autistic young people that I have worked with had said how confusing it is when adults use expressions like 'just put it there' without a clear indication of where 'there' is. Instead, it is better to say, 'put it on the blue chair'. Similarly, adults can be very vague with time language, e.g. 'we are going later' with no clear information about what later actually means or when that is. The fourth parental perspective in Chapter 2 highlighted this when talking about her daughter's understanding of language:

On repeatedly becoming distressed when hearing people use the word 'really' to indicate surprise or doubt (as opposed to 'really fast' or 'really big'), I came to realise that her understanding of language is very concrete, to the extent that significant proportions of conversation are incomprehensible to her.

- We often see Autistic children with stronger spoken language than understanding of language; this can lead to adults overestimating what a child can understand. Children can also look like they understand when they are masking.

Tip

We can support understanding and processing of language by:

- Using clear and direct language
- Getting down to a child's level and saying their name
- Breaking instructions down into chunks
- Observing them to make sure that they have understood

- **Differences with joint attention** which we have talked about already.
- **Difficulties with using and understanding non-verbal communication:** This may include facial expressions, tone, volume and rate of speech, body language and touching as well as gestures. The fourth parent perspective in Chapter 2 summarised this really clearly and the examples highlight how stressful non-verbal communication can be when it is hard to understand:

  When she was 5 years old and another mum put a bag of duck food out, to offer my daughter to take some, I realised she didn't understand basic gestures. On her asking me why I was angry when I was concentrating or confused, I came to realise that she struggles to read facial expressions.

- **Differences in social language and communication style:** This is discussed more in Chapter 5. A key reminder: social interaction and communication in Autistic children is different but not wrong!
- **Difficulties with expressing needs and preferences and self-advocacy**: In my experience this is really difficult for Autistic children of all ages and can result in both meltdowns and shutdowns. Being able to express your needs and advocate for yourself is a really important tool.

It is important to not underestimate the impact of the environment and how this can affect communication in Autistic children. A supportive and predictable environment can make a child feel safe and secure and communication will be easier. Conversely, sensory overwhelm, changes to the routine with no warning, anxiety and masking are all factors that have a big impact on a child's ability to communicate. We need to tune into environmental factors and consider the impact this will have.

I work with a little boy who had a very close bond with his key worker. Recently the key worker was on a training course for three days. Unfortunately this was not communicated to the parents, so it was not possible to prepare him for the change. He came into nursery and there was a different key worker who didn't consistently use the visuals and strategies he was familiar with. He 'held it together all day' but became very distressed after nursery. The parents had to do some detective work to understand what had happened. A simple discussion around the environmental change could have prevented this as well as better home/school communication using a home/school notebook.

What can we do to help?

We now turn to consider how we can help Autistic children to build their communication skills. Like many of the strategies outlined in this manual, this also echoes the principle of 'change yourself not the child'. If we adapt our communication, we can support Autistic children. We are not looking to change a child or reduce particular forms of communication. The aim of supporting communication is to reduce frustration and provide a child with tools to enable them to partake in activities that motivate them. When we talk about communication it is important to recognise that frustration and protesting are also a natural part of communication that all children need and should be allowed to express. For many Autistic children this may be through crying, shouting or behaviours. We are not reducing frustration to get compliance; reducing frustration is about supporting. More on this later in this chapter when we talk about autonomy and self-advocacy!

Remember, communication is much more than words. Many of the activities we now discuss are not focussing specifically on 'talking'. Supporting joint attention and non-verbal communication helps to lay important foundation skills for a child. You can help parents understand this by explaining that we are working on 'communication fundamentals'. Often 'not talking' is one of the main things parents are worried about in their children. There is sometimes a tendency to focus on teaching a child using flash cards or focussing on descriptive words such as colours and numbers. Whilst these activities do have their place, it is important to develop all of a child's communication rather than just measuring progress through words learnt.

Tip

Sometimes having lots of advice from different professionals is overwhelming. It can feel like there is a lot to do! Remember, communication is everywhere! You don't need to have a special time of day to carry out these activities, and many can be built into your everyday routines.

Using Alternative and Augmentative Communication

Alternative and Augmentative Communication (AAC) refers to any tools or strategies that help a child communicate when they are not consistently using spoken language. The aim of introducing and using AAC is to reduce frustration and support a child's ability to participate. AAC is affirmative and builds on the perspective that 'communication is a human right' and is not reliant on spoken abilities. AAC also aligns with the principle that just because a child might not speak using words it does not mean that they don't have anything to say. When I first qualified as an SLT, we tended to use the picture exchange communication system (PECS) for children at early stages of communication. PECS is not considered an affirmative approach to support Autistic children and would not be recommended. Since that time, the evidence and knowledge that SLTs have around AAC use in Autistic children has developed and shifted. Use of AAC has increased significantly and this has been really positive.

AAC is typically divided into two different types:

Unaided AAC – does not rely on any physical things and could be signing, facial expressions or body language.

Aided AAC – can be paper based (this encompasses anything not electrical including communication boards, books and objects of reference) or it can be powered, e.g. a specific communication aid or device with an AAC app.

AAC can help children:

- Reduce frustration
- Build language
- Build social connections
- By not stopping speech development

AAC is often part of a total communication approach where a child may be using words, vocalisations and have a communication book. AAC is typically introduced by an SLT working with a child and it is important to seek advice around this for any child you are working with to ensure that the right AAC is selected. This is particularly important when introducing a powered device. Lot of families I have met have downloaded a communication app that hasn't been set up properly for their child and as a result it is not seen as helpful. Working with an SLT to support AAC use is important. In most areas there is an NHS service that can provide support and advice around introducing AAC and in many areas more specialist powered devices can be funded.

Whilst AAC should always be introduced with support from an SLT, the following provides a list of key tips that can be used to support children with AAC.

The following websites are very helpful with lots of information and training resources. The Ace Centre has many free downloadable AAC resources including many nursery specific core boards:

https://acecentre.org.uk
https://www.assistiveware.com
https://thinksmartbox.com

Principles in supporting Autistic children using AAC

- **Model language:** Model language using the AAC, do not test or prompt. Modelling of AAC is one of the most important principles. It's important to focus on core words (important vocabulary) for the child and match the child's language level. This means that you need to point to the symbols as you speak. By modelling you are showing a child how to use AAC in their natural routines. Avoid prompting, 'show me what you want for snack', or using any hand over hand prompting.
- **Ensure AAC is accessible:** Make sure the AAC is accessible throughout the day; it is important that it is not only available to the child at certain times chosen by the adult.
- **Respect and acknowledge all forms of communication:** AAC supports communication, it does not replace other forms. AAC users will likely use a range of different forms of communication, and it is important to respond and acknowledge all forms.
- **Collaborate and communicate:** Work closely with the child's family and SLT.

- **Value autonomy:** AAC is more than just requesting, a child needs to have access to a range of communication functions, and it is important that these are listened to and acknowledged. AAC users need to be able to say no, protest, express preferences, comment and share preferences.
- If a child uses a powered device consider what you call it. Don't just say 'get the IPAD or AAC', often we use the word 'talker' as it is associated with being the child's voice. Talk to parents about this so you have a consistent way to describe a device.

Using core boards

Core boards are frequently used in the early years environment to support communication in Autistic children. These are pictures but they are different from visual timetables. Understanding the difference between visuals to support understanding (such as visual timetables and first/then boards) and visuals that support expression (including all forms of AAC) is really important. A core board is a type of AAC that shows 'core words' in a predictable way to support different functions of communication, it can be paper or digital. Core words are words that we use all the time in a lot of different situations. They are useful and motivating and don't just focus on requesting. On the board the pictures stay in the same place at all times so that they support memory. As mentioned, the Ace Centre website provides many free downloadable core boards which are worth having a look at.

The adult models the language whilst pointing to the pictures. For example, with a core board for bubbles there would be a range of words, e.g. bubbles, more, stop, pop, blow, like it, uh oh, look. You can create and model lots of different word combinations to narrate the child's play. For example, if the child wants more bubbles you can point to and say, 'more bubbles', 'blow', 'I like it' and then when they pop, 'pop pop pop, uh oh'. Using core boards helps to teach flexible language and not just requesting. Core boards help Autistic children who have a GLP language learning style. They are visual which supports a child's processing of language.

Core boards can help Autistic children in the following ways:

- With expressing likes/dislikes as well as asking for things
- Supporting children to combine words
- Reducing pressure to find the right words
- Supporting connection
- Generating new language

Helping a child to have their needs met

We want to help children to develop a range of language, not just requesting or asking for things. However, not being able to have your needs met can cause frustration and distress. It is therefore important to consider how we can help children to have their needs met, both through building skills and also adapting the environment around them. I often see children who are considered 'behavioural' or having a meltdown simply because they are unable to communicate what they need. I also see children who don't ask for the things they need at all for a range of reasons. When I visit a child in an education environment, I ask staff working with the child and the child's parents, 'How does he ask for things?' or 'How does she tell you which one she wants?' I am never surprised by the responses; often staff working with a child may say, 'He doesn't really ask', or 'She is so independent.... she just gets everything herself'. Parents tend to respond, 'We know what he wants so he doesn't really need to ask'. Naturally everything may be available to a child so they may not need to ask.

Imagine yourself in a foreign country – if you couldn't speak the language, one of the first things you would learn to communicate would be to tell others your basic needs. In the same way, Autistic children will be most motivated to communicate what they want. Supporting a child to ask for things and have their needs met helps to reduce frustration; it can also help with their confidence as well as building connection and trust. A child can make requests verbally, non-verbally and through AAC. It is also important to remember that requesting is only part of communication, and we need to be using strategies that support flexible language development as described earlier.

Recognising that you can do a lot to help a child ask for things is important. This can be extremely powerful for a child, as illustrated by Jack's case study.

Case study: supporting Jack in asking for things and making requests

We talked about supporting Jack's understanding in Chapter 3. Let's recap and look at how staff working with Jack supported his ability to make requests.

Background

Jack started nursery at age two and a half; at this time, he was non-speaking and did not consistently respond to spoken words. The environment was very overwhelming for him, and he would become upset whenever an adult attempted to direct him onto an activity or take him to change his nappy or wash hands. He loved the cars and would focus on these intently lying down watching them at eye level. Jack spent a lot of time doing this. Staff working with him were keen to help him engage more so that he could access new and different learning opportunities and reduce his frustration. Jack was unable to ask for anything and would communicate by screaming and pushing items away. He occasionally took an adult's hand to lead to the area where he wanted something and would reach towards a preferred item. Often Jack would climb to reach what he wanted and become frustrated when unable to communicate this to those around him.

Difficulty in making his needs known to others

Jack has difficulties with 'asking'. He is beginning to understand that he can send a message to another person, for example, by taking his or her hand or reaching towards something. Most of the time he tries to get what he wants, and when he can't he becomes upset. The impact of this is significant; Jack can become distressed when unable to tell others what he wants. People around Jack sometimes misunderstand his communication and think he is having a tantrum or 'being difficult'.

What can we do to help?

Jack needs his communication partners to tune into how he communicates. It is important that they understand more about his motivations and preferences so that they can naturally tune into him.

Change yourself, not the child

By changing the environment, as described in Chapter 3, and also changing how we communicate with young Autistic children we can make a big impact.

Actions

Staff got to know Jack and completed the iceberg (I:1) and information gathering tools (I:2). From this they were able to identify his profile of strengths and needs. Staff met with Jack's parents to discuss how they could best support him. Parents and staff agreed on the following targets for Jack. Alongside these all staff working with

Jack needed to learn more about how and why he communicates and tune into these so as to understand him better.

Targets

- For adults to create chances for Jack to communicate.
- For Jack to reach for a favourite object when offered a choice
- For Jack to 'give' an item to ask for help
- For Jack to vocalise for 'go' as part of ready, steady, go game

Strategies used

Staff working with Jack consistently used the following strategies:

- Offering choices of preferred and non-preferred snacks and toys (C:4)
- Making chances for Jack to give items in play activities
- As described in Chapter 3, focussing on using consistent language – language for routines (E:8), which meant that Jack was frequently hearing repeated words and phrases that were meaningful to him
- Helping Jack understand the concept of 'finished' (E:4)
- Because this particular group of staff were quite musical, introducing a routine song for different activities including tidying up, snack time, shoes on off, as well as showing an object

The results

In three months, Jack is more confident in making his needs known, he is sending intentional messages to others and staff have noticed his cheeky sense of humour. He does not yet communicate using words but is much less frustrated as he is clearly able to send a message in a number of ways:

- Jack is able to make a choice by reaching; he also makes a sound to indicate the item he wants.
- Jack consistently gives items to show that he wants them. For example, he will give an adult the bubbles when he wants an adult to blow them. Jack loves musical toys, but he can't start the wind-up toy on his own, so now knows to give it to an adult to play. He will make a sound for 'go'.

Self-advocacy and autonomy

In this book so far, we have talked about the neurodiversity paradigm and the importance of hearing and listening to Autistic voices. We also need to really listen to the children we work with and start building skills around self-advocacy and autonomy. I regularly work with older Autistic children and teens on self-advocacy and recognise it is vital to start early. Supporting young children with self-advocacy and autonomy is really important in early years and builds foundation skills for being able to do this as you get older.

Figure 4.1 summarises examples of self-advocacy and autonomy in children in early years. Self-advocacy at this stage is about allowing children choice and not expecting compliance.
It is important to recognise that many children will not be able to do this verbally. Self-advocacy may look like a child playing alone, shouting 'NO' or pushing something away.

Can you think of any more examples?

We can support children with the following strategies and guiding principles, many of these should be familiar terms and ideas to you by now:

- Honor and respond to all forms of communication. You can model language around preferences and autonomy, e.g. instead of saying 'use your words' you can model 'I don't like it' and acknowledge you know they don't like it.

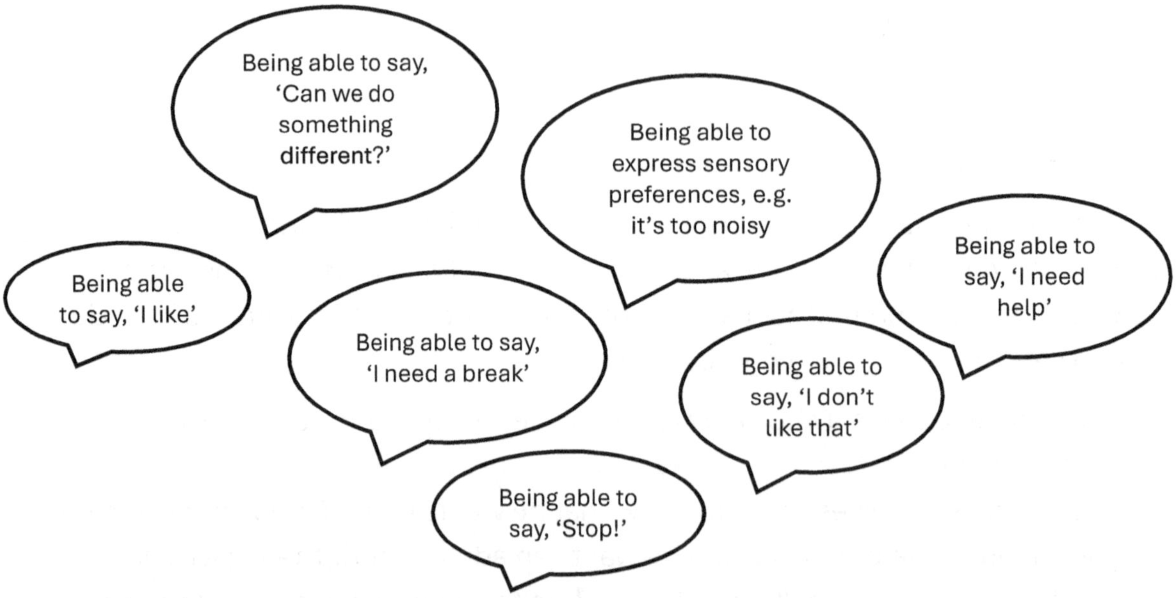

Figure 4.1 Examples of self-advocacy and autonomy

- Offer and respond to the choices Autistic children make. Offer lots of different choices throughout the day. This helps to build agency.
- Teach words like 'no' and 'stop' as well as modelling useful phrases such as 'I don't like it'.
- Model language around sensory preferences, e.g. 'it's too noisy', 'it's too bright', 'I don't like that smell', etc. You can describe what a child is doing, e.g. you are covering your ears, let's get headphones.
- Use core words within AAC that support self-advocacy, e.g. 'help', 'stop', 'break', 'all done', 'different' and 'I want'.
- Don't place demands, e.g. prompts to 'say it' or prompts to 'look at me'.
- Model language around taking breaks and provide access to a range of breaks, e.g. a quiet break, a movement break, snack, etc. Helping a child learn that they may need different breaks at different times is helpful.
- Use visuals where possible to support with this. I have made children 'self-advocacy cards' that the adult can model in the situations. It is important to personalise these, e.g. 'it's too noisy', 'can we go?', 'I want to go'. I recently made a series of self-advocacy cards with a young person at age ten. They have been really powerful for him and allow him to advocate for himself; he has really enjoyed the process of making and using them. He has created many cards, but examples include 'I need to leave now', 'don't touch me', 'please don't shorten my name, I don't like it', 'I am close to exploding'.

We will turn now to consider specific activities to support communication skills in Autistic children in activity sheets (C:1)–(C:16).

A few things not to do ... Ever!

- Don't withhold items. Whilst we want to create opportunities to support a child to communicate, we do not ever want to withhold.
- Don't say 'use your words'! I hear this all the time.
- Don't prize words above other forms of communication.
- Don't interpret protesting and saying 'no' as behaviour; Autistic children need opportunities to be autonomous.

C:1 Communication activity sheet 1. Developing joint and shared attention

C:1

Joint and shared attention are building blocks of communication. Remember that these skills can look different in Autistic children. The following strategies are repeated here from earlier in the chapter.

Affirming ways to develop joint and shared attention

- Autistic children will need to connect with you before sharing attention. Tuning into their preferences and interests is very important to support this.
- Follow a child's lead and interest.
- Join with their interest rather than trying to impose your activity.
- Make comments rather than asking questions.
- Accept all forms of showing and sharing.
- Remove pressure for eye contact.
- Joint attention will grow best in situations where there are not high demands, where there is low pressure and we are following a child's interests and preferences.

What skills are you looking for?

Working on joint attention can feel abstract; here are some of the skills you may see in a child as they start to develop:

- A shared focus – looking at the same activity as you
- Responding when you look or point at something
- Pointing or looking at items to share interest
- Showing you things that are interesting to them (not asking you for them)

Remember that these may not be accompanied by eye contact in the same way that neurotypical children may do.

Activities to develop joint attention

- Join a child warmly in their choice of activity, follow their lead and don't direct. This could be in any activity that is motivating to them.
- Have an exciting bag of motivating objects that you take out and show the child. These may be light-up toys, bubbles or whatever is motivating to the child. You are looking for the child to join the activity for a short period. Resist the temptation to try and get them to show other skills, such as requesting.

- Put items in unusual places, for example, a big sticker on the window, or a favourite toy on the shelf. Use the word 'Look!' Emphasise your pointing to direct their attention to activities. Don't expect the child to then look back at you. It needs to feel realistic.
- Make a shared focus fun and exciting and use your facial expressions and props to engage the child.
- Use materials with motivating sensory properties, for example, pouring sand, water, shaking, shredded paper and so on. Consider what an individual child likes and tailor your activities to these.

Materials needed

- Dependent on individual child

C:2 Communication activity sheet 2. The power of pausing

C:2

Pausing is a powerful way to support communication. This is especially important for children with emerging communication skills. When children don't communicate much, there is a tendency to overcompensate and talk a lot for them. By stepping back and pausing, we offer valuable opportunities for connection.

When we pause, we give a child...

- Time to process
- A chance to communicate
- Greater opportunities for connection

Activity sheets (C:4) to (C:8) all incorporate pausing as part of the strategies used.

When you pause during an activity...

- Get down to the child's level
- Be engaged – use your facial expression and gestures to show a child that you are pausing expectantly for him or her to respond. Rather than waiting with a neutral face, communicate to the child that you are waiting excitingly for something to happen. Imagine being a young child, and it is Christmas tomorrow. Think about how your face may appear!
- Pause at a key point during the activity
- Think about what you want the child to do; for example, are you looking for him or her to communicate with you that he or she wants more? Remember to respond to all of a child's attempts to communicate; this may be looking, body movements or sounds.
- Remember there is no pressure on the child to do anything. You are pausing to give him or her a chance to connect and also to see how they respond.

Tip

Practise your pausing face! By putting in pauses to our communication, we also slow down what we are saying and become more conscious of how and why we are communicating and interacting with a child.

C:3 Communication activity sheet 3. Imitation 'copy me'!

C:3

Imitation is a powerful communication strategy to use, especially with children at early stages of communication. Imitation is a key part of an approach called intensive interaction (Hewett, 2011**) that is frequently used with Autistic children and adults. It is definitely worth looking up the approach to find out more about it.**

Think of when you hold a little baby. He or she makes a sound, and we naturally coo back. Imitation is a natural way of supporting communication. The great thing is that you can do it anywhere and don't need any resources at all. Sometimes you can feel a little self-conscious; however, the more you can commit and be at the child's level, the more powerful your imitation will be.

Through imitating a child's sounds and actions, we are helping him or her understand that his or her communication is powerful and has an impact on other people.

For more information on intensive interaction, see www.intensiveinteraction.org

Through imitating a child, we can help a child to...

- Connect joyfully
- Have a shared focus
- Take simple turns in an activity
- Learn to imitate you (although this is not the goal)
- Engage with you in a non-pressured way

How to imitate

- Start off by watching the child – what is he or she interested in?
- Join the child in the activity rather than trying to get him or her to do your activity
- Be face to face
- Follow his or her interests and what he or she is doing
- Copy sounds and actions
- Pause to see how the child responds
- Keep the interaction going – make it fun

- Remember there is no pressure for the child to 'do anything' in particular. You are providing an opportunity for shared focus and time to communicate.
- You may feel silly to start with, but it is worth making the effort

How to step it up

- Once you have established a shared focus, try adding in something new.

Materials needed

- None

C:4 Communication activity sheet 4. Making chances to communicate – offering choices

C:4

Offering choices is a useful way to help children make requests and create opportunities for them to make their needs known. By offering a choice we can help a child to show what he or she wants and reduce frustration. Choice making provides an opportunity for modelling language and ways for a child to communicate such as reaching, pointing and looking. By offering choices to children who have language, we are reducing the number of direct questions we ask and providing an opportunity to model new language. Offering choices also builds autonomy and self-advocacy.

How to offer choices

- Start off by offering a choice between motivating and un-motivating items; that is, offer the child a choice between what he or she wants and something he or she is less interested in. This means that the child will communicate what he or she wants rather than reaching for both or losing interest.
- Clearly say what each option is; for example, say, 'Do you want ball or book?' whilst holding each item forward. This means that the child is hearing the single word whilst hearing the object.
- Your child may choose by looking, reaching, making a sound or using the word to communicate which one he or she wants.
- As soon as the child indicates which item he or she wants, give it immediately, saying the name of the object he or she chose.

When to offer choices

You can offer choices at any time of day! In nursery this can be a good strategy to use consistently at certain times of the day, for example, snack time, song choosing during circle time or before going out to the playground. You can offer choices using objects or pictures if the objects are not immediately available. When there are lots of options it can be helpful to make it visual and use a choosing board (C:9).

How to step it up

- Choice making is a useful strategy to use even when children can tell you what they would like.

- You can offer choices including new and different concepts. This gives the opportunity to hear new words and also to practise saying them. For example, if you are working on size concepts, 'Would you like a *big* apple or a *little* apple?'
- Remember, as a child develops his or her language, you can use choices in relation to different words and actions (see C:12); for example, if you are targeting a child's use of action words, try 'Shall we kick or throw the ball?'

Materials needed

- No resources needed to offer verbal choices, just the objects you are choosing between. For more choices, use a choosing board or drawing out options on a whiteboard.

C:5 Communication activity sheet 5. Making chances to communicate – giving

C:5

Typically, young children will give an item as a way of getting an adult's help or attention. This is a powerful way of communicating with those around you that you need something. Autistic children may find this harder, and it could lead to frustration; for example, if a child wanted something and the lid was on too tight, but they were unable to send a message to another person that they needed help. By supporting a child's ability to give objects we can reduce frustration.

Creating chances for Autistic children to give is an easy way to facilitate a child's ability to have their needs met. This is a great strategy as it is easy to implement and can be used effectively for children at early stages of communication. I am never not surprised at how quickly this can work. Often, I meet children and their parents say that they don't give. After modelling a few times with something highly motivating, the child starts to give the item and it creates a lovely moment of connection. It is really important to note that this is not about an adult using hand over hand prompting to give, or guiding them to give, we are merely creating a joyful opportunity in a non-pressured interaction with lots of adult support.

How to encourage children to give items

- Be face to face and at their level, think about activities the child really enjoys that may fit with this. I find blowing up a balloon and letting it go a really fun one for this; either blow it with your mouth or use a balloon pump, let the balloon blow up, then pause and let it go. Often a child (if they like the game) will run to get it; have your hand outstretched and be at their level and they may give it to you to do the game again.
- Another good one is with snacks; instead of automatically opening the container give it to the child, be nearby with your hand outstretched and model 'open' as soon as they push it towards you.
- Accept all communication forms and respond warmly.

Example: giving bubbles

1 Blow a few bubbles to get the child's interest. Make it fun; pop them to get his or her interest and engagement. Use the bubbles core board alongside it.
2 Put the lid on the bubbles too tight so that the child will be unable to open them.
3 Place the bubbles nearby and pause.

4 Offer your outstretched hand as a cue. When the child gives you the bubbles, say 'bubbles' or model 'blow bubbles' or 'more bubbles' and immediately blow them.

Why would we say bubbles rather than thank you or more? It is much better to teach the child the word for the object rather than a more abstract term, particularly for children with limited language. This is a really nice activity to use a core board in to ensure that we are modelling a range of words and communicative functions as well as supporting the child to give it to you.

When to practise giving

Try this at any time of the day, although avoid times of tiredness or frustration. Remember we never want to be withholding items.

Materials needed

- Clear plastic boxes
- Motivating toys and objects

C:6 Communication activity sheet 6. Making chances to communicate – a bit at a time

C:6

Naturally as parents and educators, we want to meet children's needs. For example, if we know that children like raisins, it makes sense to give them a bowl of raisins at snack time. We want them to be happy and enjoy the raisins. But we can make many everyday activities into an opportunity for communication by offering things a little at a time. Instead of giving everything all at once, give a few pieces and wait to see how a child asks you for more. This pausing also creates opportunity for commenting and shared connection. Depending on the level of communication, a child may reach, point, make a sound or say a word to communicate with you that he or she wants more. Again, use of a snack core board alongside this would be helpful.

This strategy works well in the following activities

With all these activities you can use a core board to model other functions of language and make the activity visual.

Snacks

- Instead of leaving snacks out, offer a few pieces at a time. Keep snacks in a Tupperware container. This also encourages giving (C:5).

Puzzles

- Use a plastic wallet with a zip to keep puzzles in. Offer a few pieces and wait to see how the child 'asks' you for more. Remember to model a range of language, e.g. 'I like it', 'it's fun'.

Train tracks

- Keep hold of a few pieces of train track and wait to see how the child 'asks' you for more.Activity Think about what other activities in your environment lend themselves to offering a bit at a time.

Materials needed

- Toys
- Plastic boxes and wallets
  - Core boards and visual resources

C:7 Communication activity sheet 7. Ready, steady, go games

C:7

Playing ready, steady, go games can be a useful way to get a child to send you a message that he or she wants the game to start or carry on. Ready, steady, go creates predictable play routines and opportunities for joyful connection.

How to play a ready, steady, go game

- Think about an activity that the child may find motivating. Start with a game that he or she already enjoys.
- Start the game, for example, blowing a few bubbles or building a tower.
- Use facial expressions and tone to create interest and excitement.
- Say, 'Ready, steady ... (pause before the exciting bit happens, then say) go'.
- Pause and wait expectantly to give the child a chance to request.
- Remember to wait expectantly and excitedly!
- Respond to any attempt to communicate made by the child, for example, looking, reaching or making a sound.

You can incorporate ready, steady, go into lots of favourite games

Bubbles: Instead of blowing the bubbles continuously, blow a few bubbles. Wait and say, 'Ready, steady ... go!' Wait for the child to show you how he or she wants you to blow the bubbles. He or she may move closer, reach, make a sound or look. Repeat several times and honour all communication attempts. Remember this is also about creating connection and joy.

On the swing: Pull the swing back, and say, 'Ready, steady ... go'! Wait for your child to show you how he or she wants you to release the swing. He or she may wriggle, vocalise or try to say 'go'.

Knocking over a tower: Slowly build a tower either together or with the child watching you in anticipation. Say, 'Ready, steady ... go'! Repeat several times.

Pull back cars and wind-up toys: The advantage of these toys is that they can be hard to operate so that the child may give you them as well to start the game (C:3).Activity Think of children you work with. What could you use as a ready, steady, go game with them?

Materials needed

- Toys to use as part of the ready, steady, go game

C:8 Communication activity sheet 8. Stop/go games

The principles of a stop/go game are similar to ready, steady, go games (C:7). Stop/go games can be highly motivating for children and also provide an opportunity for them to be in control and use their communication and be listened to. I have seen children with significant communication difficulties initiate go by moving their bodies and smiling or gently raising their hand. We can respond to all attempts to communicate. These are motivating activities that also provide a great opportunity for joint attention (C:1).

How to play a stop/go game

- Decide what you are going to stop/go. This will depend on the child's motivation and interest.
- Start the game, for example, shaking the parachute, saying 'ready, steady, go' ... pausing, and saying, 'stop'. Hold your hands up in a gesture to show 'stop'.
- Say 'ready, steady ... go' and wait for the child to start the activity again (as outlined in C:5).
- Use facial expressions and tone to create interest and excitement.
- Pause and wait expectantly to give the child a chance to request.
- Remember to wait expectantly and excitedly! To start off, you may need to wait for at least five to ten seconds.
- Respond to any attempt to communicate made by the child, for example, looking, reaching and making a sound.
- Be consistent in your words and gestures that you use as part of the game. Repetition will help a child learn the steps of the game.

Ideas for stop/go games

Pouring: Pouring can be highly visual and motivating for some children. Use a stop/go game when pouring water at the water table or sand at the sand tray. Get creative and think about what else you can pour, for example, rice onto a tray or coloured water onto a tray.

Shaking a parachute: Parachutes are a great resource to use for lots of activities.

Shaking a tinfoil blanket: I use tinfoil blankets a lot as part of games, firstly because they are extremely cheap and durable, and secondly they add a level of excitement and motivation for children who like sensory play. They make a great noise and visual display. Either sit the child you are working with on the blanket and shake/stop around him or her or get him or her to hold the blanket and be involved in shaking.

Musical instruments: where the child can communicate stop and go for the activity. I recently used these with an older child using drums using her AAC. She really enjoyed telling me to stop/go using her talker and this was a powerful way I could listen to her voice.

How to step it up

For children who are learning more language, add in concepts; for example, 'Shall we go fast/slow, high/low (shaking blanket)?' Be creative. Remember to keep language to the child's level.

Materials needed

- Toys to use as part of the stop/go game

C:9 Communication activity sheet 9. Making choices with a choosing board

C:9

(C:4) outlines the importance of offering choices. Choice making is an easy strategy to incorporate into the environment to help children to make requests throughout the day. Often it is relatively easy to use the real objects when making a choice, for example, snack items or choosing different-coloured paper in a craft activity. Sometimes it can be harder to have all the items there to choose from. On these occasions it may be useful to use a choosing board.

What is a choosing board?

Using a choosing board is a helpful way to offer choices when there are lots of options. They work well when the choices feel overwhelming and there are too many to list verbally. They work well for songs, playground, snack, game choice, choosing a friend, etc., with the caveat that there is always the option for the child to say 'no'.

See Figure 4.2 for an example (this is line drawings for the purposes of illustrating here but symbols or photographs of real items are better).

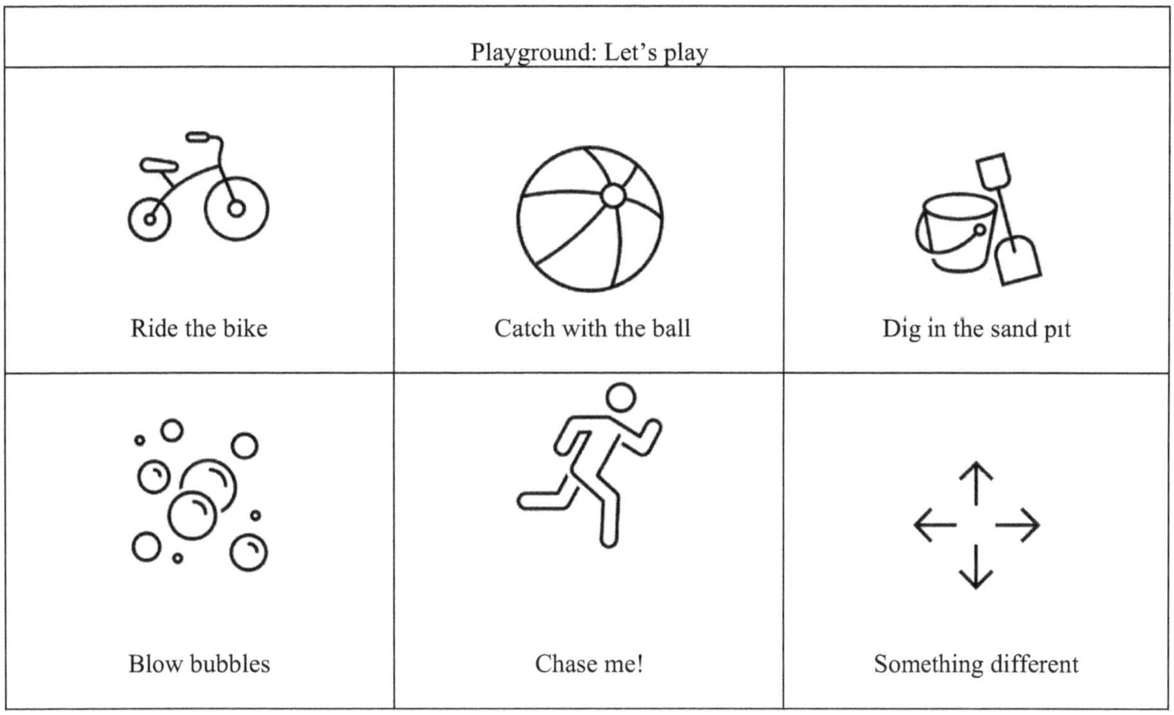

Figure 4.2 Example choice board

How to use

- Offer the child the board – keep your language consistent; for example, 'let's play ... catch the ball', 'let's play ... dig in the sand'. Point to each picture as you say each option. Your language can be more or less, depending on the child. Remember to also model other language, e.g. if they choose the bike you could model 'I love bikes', or 'let's go fast'.
- Remember autonomy and self-advocacy and always include a way for the child to be saying 'none of these', or 'something different'.

Materials needed

- Photos or symbols
- Laminator

C:10 Communication activity sheet 10. Asking for help

C:10

Being able to ask for help is an incredibly useful tool and something that many Autistic children find hard. Often it is something I support in older primary and secondary children, therefore providing support now is important. Children may request help in a variety of ways, for example, by bringing you an item that he or she can't operate by giving it to you or just by standing near you. Some children may not ask for help at all, and others may throw an item.

As a first step we need to be really tuned into the children we work with, so we are able to model asking for help as much as possible. We can also adapt the environment and create chances to enable children to successfully ask for help.

We need to create chances for a child to ask for help. This very much draws on the strategies outlined in (C:2)–(C:5). If we are able to set up these opportunities, we can support a child in asking for help in whatever way they need. Remember the way that a child asks you for help will depend on his or her verbal level. For example, a child at early stages of communication may just stand near you or give you the item, whereas a child with more language may say, 'Help', or 'Help, please'. Often there can be a mismatch in that children who are fluent communicators may really find communicative functions like asking for help really hard.

How to create chances to ask for help

- Model asking for help throughout daily routines, e.g. putting on boots, shoes, etc. Use clear language related to asking for help, e.g. if you see a child struggling to reach something don't just reach up, get it for them and say 'here you go', as you've missed a chance to model asking for help. Model language from the child's perspective, e.g. 'I need help', 'help me please'.
- When creating opportunities to ask for help use motivating activities for a child that align with his or her interests.
- Make a chance for him or her to communicate, for example, by putting the lid on too tight or putting a favourite toy slightly out of reach. Toys that are harder to operate also create a good opportunity, e.g. a wind-up toy or spin toy. Remember: gently creating opportunities is helpful, intentionally witholding items is not.
- When they try to do it themselves, offer a cue; for example, extend an outstretched hand and say, 'I need help' or 'help me'.

- Pause and wait to see how the child asks you; this may be by giving you the item. Continue to model language around asking for help.
- Don't ask the child to repeat you or say, 'say help me, please'. Don't ask questions such as 'do you need help?', particularly for GLP language learners – this is unhelpful. Remember to use declarative language when modelling (from the child's perspective).

When to ask for help

Asking for help can be tailored to a range of activities. Easy ones within the early years environment include snack time or play activities. This is never about withholding items or causing frustration.

Materials needed

- Toys that are motivating but too hard for children to operate themselves

C:11 Communication activity sheet 11. Using songs

C:11

In Chapter 3, we talked about how we can use songs to support understanding of routines. Music can be a powerful motivator, and we know that GLP language learners often love music and learn music through songs. Songs and singing also create a lovely opportunity for shared joy and connection. As well as just singing the songs we can use strategies to increase predictability and support communication using the following strategies.

How to use songs to support communication

- **Start the song the same way** – Use a consistent gesture, word or action. You may add a visual cue such as an object or symbol; for example, say, 'Row, row', show the boat and put your hands outstretched.
- **Be face to face** – Being at a child's level is important to support communication. This might mean sitting or lying on the floor. It also means that you can see all of the child's attempts to communicate with you; you are then ideally placed to respond straightaway.
- **Respond to and interpret all of a child's attempts to communicate** – This may be eye contact, a wiggle, a smile or a sound. When you respond immediately and continue the song, this helps a child learn about sending messages to make things happen.
- **Pause during key points** – In (C:2) we talked about how pausing and waiting is an important strategy as it gives a child the opportunity to ask for more. A child may ask for more by looking at you, reaching for your hands or vocalizing. Pause during exciting parts of the song, for example, in 'Row, Row, Row Your Boat' just before the scream. Pause and wait to see if a child fills in the sound or word.
- **Incorporate movement and props to create anticipation** – During 'Zoom Zoom' after five, four, three, two, one, lift your child up, pause and create anticipation.
- **Think about how the child you are working with is going to ask you for more and offer cues to help this** – In 'Round and Round the Garden Like a Teddy Bear', pause and offer your hand. Your child may reach for your hand to communicate he or she wants more. As he or she becomes used to the routine, he or she may reach for your hand and make a sound or use a word.
- **Make it visual** – Use objects of reference or a choice board to allow the child to choose the song. Then use a core board alongside singing. A core board can provide opportunities for a child to express preferences around more, stop, louder, quieter,

faster, slower, change the song, I like it, I don't like it as well as other actions, e.g. let's dance!

Activity

Think of a child and a song that he or she likes. Use the following checklist to break the song down to support communication:

- How will you start the song; for example, with a sound, word and/or gesture?
- How will you create chances to communicate; for example, pause at an exciting point?
- How will you finish the song?

How to step it up

For children who regularly join in songs, you could add choices with different concepts; for example, 'Shall we sing loud or quiet/fast or slow?'

Materials needed

- Objects or pictures to represent songs or choice board
- Core boards – see Ace Centre website (https://acecentre.org.uk)

C:12 Communication activity sheet 12. Adding language

C:12

Even when children aren't talking, they are often listening and learning language. Being able to add language to your activities and interaction is a helpful way to support understanding and expression. SLTs often call this 'modelling language' and we know that it is a very powerful strategy. We need to model language at the right level that is flexible and functional, not just labelling nouns. I had a session recently with an OT and specialist teacher with a five-year-old Autistic boy who had recently been introduced to AAC. In the session there were lots of lovely activities, swinging, jumping, hide and seek as well as sensory play using foam (making snow). At the end of the session both the teacher and the OT commented that I talked a lot more than they normally did in the session. We discussed that whilst it is important to create a calm environment for a child and not bombard with too much language, we do need to be modelling language at the right level. They reflected that their sessions tended to be very quiet with them using minimal talking and when they did offer modelling it only tended to be around requesting, e.g. 'I want swing' or 'I want more'. We reflected that adding some more language for a wider range of functions would be really helpful for this child. Several weeks on and they are chatting more and reporting that he is using words on his talker like 'faster' and saying, 'let's play' and 'chase me'! All because of modelling more language.

Cut the questions!

- As adults we ask a lot of questions, even to children who can't necessarily respond. Instead of asking questions, you can make comments and model language to support a child's communication. SLTs talk about the hand rule: imagine holding up your hand with four fingers and a thumb, essentially for every question we ask we need to follow up with four comments. So, in play, a 4:1 comment to question ratio. (C:14) has a good example of this.

Activity

Time yourself in an interaction with a child for ten minutes and consciously count the number of questions you ask. In most cases you will be surprised it's a lot more than you think!

Tip

Turn questions into comments as summarised in Table 4.4.

Add helpful words

- Think about words that are useful for the child, for example, rather than using words without a specific meaning, such as 'that one' and 'there'. Use the specific word.
- Don't add labels – add action words (C:13).
- Add social language, for example, 'Let's play, my turn' (S:5).

Tip

'Say it as if he/she could' is a useful rule when modelling language and means that a child is exposed to more language for more functions. This also has the benefit of aligning with their interest and sense of humour! I have often found modelling phrases and words like 'That's yucky', 'That's stinky' and 'disgusting' more powerful than just labelling items.

Communicate at the child's level

- Be at a child's physical level when you are talking to him or her.
- Model language at the right level; for example, if a child is using no words and we talk in long sentences, it is too much for them to take on. For example, for a child with limited language, saying, 'let's play cars, shall we have the red one or the blue one, let's go!' doesn't give the child the language they need. Instead, be at the child's level, hold a car and say, 'Let's play'.
- Remember for children with a GLP language learning style we need to model phrases not single words.

Tip

Think about how you can turn questions into comments. See Table 4.4 for some examples and ideas. Challenge yourself to change questions into comments during times of connection and play.

Table 4.4 Changing questions into comments

Instead of asking...	*Make a comment!*
'What's that?'	'It's a big dog'
'Do you like it?'	'I love dogs'
'What's the doggy doing?'	'He's eating his bone', 'the doggy is running!'
'Is that nice?'	'Mmmmm yummy snack!'

C:13 Communication activity sheet 13. Using action words

C:13

Learning action words are an important part of language development. They are key to linking words together and making longer sentences. If a child knows lots of nouns, for example, dog, water and ball, it is difficult to link words to make a sentence, for example, dog *drinks* water. Action words are key building blocks in language. Often Autistic children have large labelling vocabularies but struggle with using everyday action words. Developing action words is an important area to focus on and is easy to build on in everyday routines and play.

Ideas and activities to try

- The great thing about action words is that they occur in everyday activities when you are 'doing things'.
- Make a verb book with photos and pictures featuring action words. You can personalise, for example, 'Leo is sleeping' or 'Yafet is eating'. These pictures will be fun and motivating to make comments on and model language throughout daily activities. Children are often more motivated by pictures of themselves.
- Use practical activities during which you make and do things, for example, cooking (mix and pour) or snack time (cut fruit, drink and eat). You can use core boards to model language around different functions.
- When you are looking at pictures in books, instead of just labelling the pictures, talk about what the people are doing.
- Try not to test your child, for example, asking, 'What are they doing?' Instead make comments at the time they are happening; for example, 'I am eating... yummy!'
- Add to and expand what the child is saying with an action word; for example, when he or she comments, 'Look, dog', you say, 'Yes, the dog is running'.
- Choose several action words to focus on each week, and comment on these in everyday activities. Remember that when learning new words, children need lots of repetition across different activities and contexts.
- Start off with everyday, common verbs, for example, eat, drink, sleep and jump, before moving onto more abstract verbs such as pull, pour, hop and so on. Choose action words that are motivating to a child, so if they love swinging and climbing these are the ones to choose.
- Use natural gestures to reinforce understanding and provide a visual cue.

- Once you feel the child understands the verbs, you can give choices in activities to help him or her use the words; for example, when playing with the ball, ask, 'Shall Mummy kick the ball or throw the ball?'

Materials needed

- Photographs (only for verb book)

C:14 Communication activity sheet 14. Supporting gestalt language processors

C:14

Earlier in this chapter we talked about the Gestalt Language Processing. This activity sheet provides a summary of tips and strategies you can use to support gestalt language processors.

Remember, all forms of communication are valid: some children learn language in chunks, and some learn language through building up single words. Our job is to understand the meaning of what a child is trying to convey and support their communication. We do not have to stop them using chunks of language. This is very important. The strategies to support gestalt language processors can be built into daily play activities and are summarised in Table 4.5.

Table 4.5 Strategies to support gestalt language processors

Strategy	*How to*
Follow a child's lead	Observe carefully then join in with a child's play rather than directing their attention onto another activity. There will be more opportunities for connection and engagement as you will be focussing on what they are interested in.
Acknowledge all communication	This is important even if you are not fully sure of the meaning or intention. You can do this non-verbally by nodding, smiling, responding warmly with your expressions and verbally by saying 'yeah' or 'ok'. Through acknowledging and responding to all communication it shows a child you are listening and encourages them to continue to communicate with you.
Model phrases	Model lots of phrases (not just single words) when children are at stages 1 and 2. This will help them move to the next stage.
Comment, narrate and use declarative language	Narrate what is happening within your daily routines. Share observations of what is happening around you. Describe what you are doing, seeing or feeling to model language as naturally as possible, such as 'I'm washing my hands' or 'It's time for lunch'. Focus on perspective: use 'I' or 'We' statements to model phrases the child can adopt, for example, saying 'Let's find it' instead of 'Go find it'.
Use fun intonation	Remember gestalt language processors tune into intonation and melody of language so making your intonation dramatic and fun will help children to pick up on your language models.
Interpret	Put into words what a child may be thinking and model this from their perspective, for example, 'I love it', 'it's so fun' or 'I don't like it'. Modelling gestalts that are meaningful to a child means they are more likely to stick.
Model language in songs	Remember gestalt language processors are often very musical. Putting words to song or singing phrases to the tune of familiar songs that your child enjoys can be helpful.

Table 4.5 (Continued)

Strategy	*How to*
Reduce questions	Focus on commenting instead of asking questions. SLTs often talk about the hand rule with a 4:1 ratio, so for every question you ask in play you need to make four comments. Reducing questions removes the pressure to provide a reply. Example of 4:1 comment ratio to questions in train play? Question: *Where is the train going?* Comments: *Look it's going under, wow it's fast, I like it, that's so funny.*
Don't take gestalts literally	We sometimes need to do detective work to figure out the intention of a gestalt. Whilst doing this remember not to take gestalts too literally.
Avoid prompting	Don't prompt with 'say....' A child is more likely to respond to more natural and spontaneous modelling of language.
Allow silences	Silences are really important to allow a child time to respond and to process what has been said. It is important to allow silences in play and other interactions.

C:15 Communication activity sheet 15. Let's create

C:15

I have always found using creative everyday activities where you 'make' something a motivating way to support language and communication skills in Autistic children. Working on an activity with a sequence gives lots of opportunities to add language (C:12) and work on action words (C:13), as well as provide opportunities for requesting (C:4–C:8) with an added bonus of providing a shared and joint focus of attention (C:1). Structured activities are also more predictable and certain, and can therefore reduce anxiety around expectations. You can use a task planner or handwritten schedule of what is going to happen as described in (E:12) to provide increased structure.

Activity ideas

- Make a sandwich or ice a biscuit.
- Make play dough – once you have made your play dough, add glitter to make it sparkly or scents.
- Prepare a snack – make a fruit salad.
- Use shaving foam to make snow, add glitter and make it sparkly snow.
- Tailor activity to the child's interests; for example, if he or she enjoys sensory exploratory play, try some of the ideas in Chapter 6 which focus on play.

Top tips

- Talk about what is happening in the order that it is happening; for example, first, then, next. Try to avoid abstract language which can change the order that things happen in, e.g. don't say after you get the bowl, 'bring the banana', as this is very confusing.
- Make it visual; you can also take photos of the activity and use it for teaching new language and sequences (C:12). The photos also are a great context for discussion and sharing what a child has been doing as part of a 'chat book'.
- Model language that is useful for each child at the right level. This can cover many communicative functions, e.g. modelling, 'I love it', 'I don't like sticky hands', 'yummy'. You may use the same activity, for example, making play dough with two different children, but your expectation of what each child will do and the language you use may be different. This goes back to the key philosophy of '*change yourself and not the child*'.

Activity

Think about making play dough with Louie and Lucille, who we met in Chapter 1. You can use the same activity with different aims and expectations for each child. What do you need to do different for each child?

Tip

Plan in advance so that you are ready for the activity; this gives more time for connection and fun! You could print the planning sheet in Table 4.6 to help you plan fun creative activities for Autistic children. Taking the time to plan needs to be a deliberate step and is important even though you may be feeling 'I don't need to do that', it means that you don't have to focus so much on what happens during the activity, leaving more time for connection, modelling language and fun. By planning consciously and deliberately we are also thinking carefully about the children we work with. Planning sheets can be kept and allow greater opportunities for consistency between adults.

Before starting, consider:

- Who is this activity for? What are they interested in? Will they like it? Sometimes as adults we can get really focussed on a really great or impressive activity that may not align with a child's sensory preferences, e.g. cornflour play for a child who doesn't like stuff on their hands is not going to be a fun 'Let's create' activity. This is about tailoring the activity to the child, not getting the child to 'fit' with the activity that you have planned.
- What do I need? Make sure you have all the materials including clear up stuff nearby.
- What strategies can I use to support the child? Think language modelling and use of core boards.
- How will I start the activity and how will I finish the activity? And what will we do next?

Remember predictability and certainty are important.

Table 4.6 Planning sheet for 'Let's create' (printable)

Let's Create Planning Sheet!	
Child's name: Date:	
Activity:	
What is the aim: personalise for the child To create shared opportunities for joy and connection. To model verbs To provide a motivating experience	
Materials needed: (materials for the activity and also support, e.g. core boards, choosing boards)	
Strategies I will use:	
How will I start the activity?	
How will I finish the activity?	
Activity observations: think about what went well; would you do anything differently next time?	
Observations: (child) include language sample	

C:16 Communication activity sheet 16. Using an about-me book or 'chat book'

C:16

Many Autistic children find it difficult to share information about themselves even if they have the language skills. Providing a context can be a great way to make this easier for them. This can be by using an about-me book. This can help a child 'offer' information about themselves, which is a good way to start conversations. For a child with developing language, he or she may like looking at the pictures with you, which can provide a shared focus and opportunity for connection.

What is an about-me book?

An about-me book, or 'chat book' as it is sometimes known, provides information and pictures about a child, his or her family, favourite toys and activities so that they have a context to share what is meaningful to them. I have worked with many Autistic children where creating such a book has provided a lovely social opportunity for connection. A little girl I worked with in a nursery really enjoyed sharing her book with all adults in the setting, including the lunch ladies and receptionist. She would not have had opportunities to connect in this way without the context of an about-me book.

How to make an about-me book

You can use an A5 folder or spiral-bound laminated sheets. Use pictures and symbols. Involve a child's parents/carers so that you can collaborate together.
The following pages are useful:

Me and my family
My favourite things
Places I like to go
I like to talk about...
Over the weekend I did...

Depending on the child's language level you could extend the book into a sharing news book in which parents stick or draw pictures of what they have done during the weekend and the same from the nursery day. All children find it difficult to answer the question, 'What did you do today?'; we know that Autistic children have strengths in their visual skills, so providing this context with pictures that are motivating to them provides a context of shared attention and connection. The book can also have lots of pictures relating to special interests to provide a context for motivating shared focus and connection.

Materials needed

- Resources to make about-me book

Chapter 4 summary

- Autistic children develop communication in a different way to neurotypical children. It therefore makes sense that Autistic children will need their communication partners to use different strategies and supports to enable them to thrive.
- Communication comes from connection; this is why joint and shared attention are important.
- Some children develop language through chunks of language and echolalia; this is known as Gestalt Language Processing. We are not looking to stop chunks of language but to support children with the right strategies so that they can move towards more flexible language use.
- We can support communication in Autistic children by making sure that there is access to Alternative and Augmentative Communication; there are many different kinds of AAC including aided, unaided, paper based and powered. A key message is that AAC does not stop children from talking and does not impact speech development.
- Core boards are a helpful way to model flexible and natural language in interaction.
- It is often difficult for Autistic children to have their needs met, to advocate for themselves and to be autonomous in their communication. As adults around them we need to change our communication to facilitate the children we work with.

References

Blanc, M. 2012. *Natural Language Acquisition on the Autism Spectrum: The Journey from Echolalia to Self-Generated Language*. Madison, WI: Communication Development Center.

Cooper, J., Moodley, M. and Reynell, J. 1978. *Helping Language Development: A Developmental Programme for Children with Early Learning Handicaps*. London: Edward Arnold.

Hewett, D. 2011. *Intensive Interaction: Theoretical Perspectives*. London: SAGE.

Prizant, B.M. 1983. Language acquisition and communicative behaviour in autism: Toward an understanding of the 'whole' of it. *Journal of Speech and Hearing Disorders*, 48(3), pp.296–307.

Prizant, B.M. and Duchan, J.F. 1981. The functions of immediate echolalia in autistic children. *Journal of Speech and Hearing Disorders*, 46, pp.241–249.

5

Social interaction

Creating a joyful connection

Chapter 5 provides the following:

- Overview of social interaction differences in Autistic children – dispelling the myths
- Guiding principles to keep in mind when supporting interaction
- Practical case studies to guide your thinking
- Tips on how to support children to participate in the social environment
- Activity sheets:
  - (S:1) – A shared social experience
  - (S:2) – A shared social focus
  - (S:3) – Making a chance to interact
  - (S:4) – Making interaction predictable by adding structure
  - (S:5) – Adding social language
  - (S:6) – Taking turns
  - (S:7) – Taking turns – making it visual
  - (S:8) – Using a turn-taking board
  - (S:9) – Let's chat – top tips for conversations
  - (S:10) – Supporting perspective taking

Social interaction in Autistic children

From the theory you have read and case studies that you have worked through so far, you know that social interaction looks different in Autistic children. You should also know by now that THAT IS OK!

DOI: 10.4324/9781003627760-5

In my work as an SLT the influence of the neurodiversity paradigm, shifting perspectives and listening to the voices of Autistic people has shifted how I talk about social communication differences in Autistic children and young people. It has also shifted how I think about support around social interaction and communication for Autistic children. Historically, when I first trained as an SLT there was a big emphasis on 'social skills' support with an aim of 'teaching' Autistic children skills to help shape their interactions with others. This is now a really outdated view; current thinking around social interaction seeks to support children and young people to connect and build tools in a way that is meaningful to them. However, there continue to be stereotypes around social interaction in Autistic children which are important to dispel. A few of these stereotypes and myths are dispelled in Table 5.1.

Table 5.1 Dispelling the myths and stereotypes around social interaction in Autistic children

Myth/stereotype	*Dispelling the myth*
'Everyone is a little bit Autistic'.	This myth is not true and very unhelpful as it is dismissive of the challenges that Autistic children experience.
Autistic children lack empathy.	This is another common myth that impacts how people understand social interaction in Autistic children. Autistic children feel emotions deeply but can find it hard to express them.
Autistic people can be rude or blunt.	This is a very common myth that I encounter! Autistic children tend to use and prefer a direct style of communication.
Autistic children need social skills training to help them have better conversations.	Conversations with Autistic children may be different and that is ok. I've learnt from the Autistic teens that I work with that 'small talk' can feel pointless and can be exhausting to engage in. Autistic children may show a preference to connect over topics of deep interest. Conversations may be different, but all forms of communication are valid.
Autistic children don't want social interaction.	This is another common but persistent myth. Autistic children very often do want social interaction and connection, but their social overtures can look different. Difficulty can come with navigating social rules, not through a lack of desire or interest. For example, a younger Autistic child may not always wave, point or show sustained eye contact but they may bring toys without eye contact, sit closely, smile and laugh during familiar play routines.
Autistic children prefer to be alone than with friends.	Another myth! Perspectives of Autistic people and relevant research studies highlight that many Autistic children feel lonely and say that they would like friends. Being excluded can cause distress. Autistic children may: • Prefer one friend rather than big groups • Enjoy structured activities rather than open-ended non-structured play • Spend time near peers rather than in conversation Sometimes this can be mistaken for disinterest but it's just a different interaction style.

Activity

Can you think of any more myths around social interaction in relation to the children you work with? Can you dispel them.

Think back to the Double Empathy Theory (Milton) from Chapter 1; this is important and helpful in breaking down stereotypes about Autism because it moves the focus from deficits sitting with the Autistic person to a view of mutual misunderstanding between Autistic and non-Autistic people. In simple terms it says, 'Autistic and non-Autistic people have different communication styles, and both may struggle to understand each other'. Keeping this in mind is a helpful way to start thinking about social interaction and how we can support Autistic children.

When we think about supporting social interaction in Autistic children, we really need to consider the premise of 'why is an Autistic child expected to learn social skills? What about everyone else learning how to communicate in ways that include them?' Essentially when we focus only on what the child needs to be doing differently in terms of teaching social skills, we overlook the responsibility of everyone else to create inclusive, supportive and responsive environments. Greater understanding and environmental changes can lead to broadening the ways that everyone connects. Often when I work with children in early years, to begin with parents are sometimes surprised that the therapy is not one on one in a different 'therapy room'. In early years my work tends to be firstly with the staff in terms of strategies they can be using and how we can adapt the environment before supporting the child directly.

Core principles

One of the parts of my work I love the most is building connection with Autistic children and young people. I keep the following core principles in mind; whilst this is not an exhaustive list it is a good starting point. You might come up with more in your own practice!

These core principles are relevant to all Autistic children; discussion of each principle is summarised next:

Accept all forms of communication:

- This may include gestalts and echolalia.
- Communication may be physical as well as verbal.

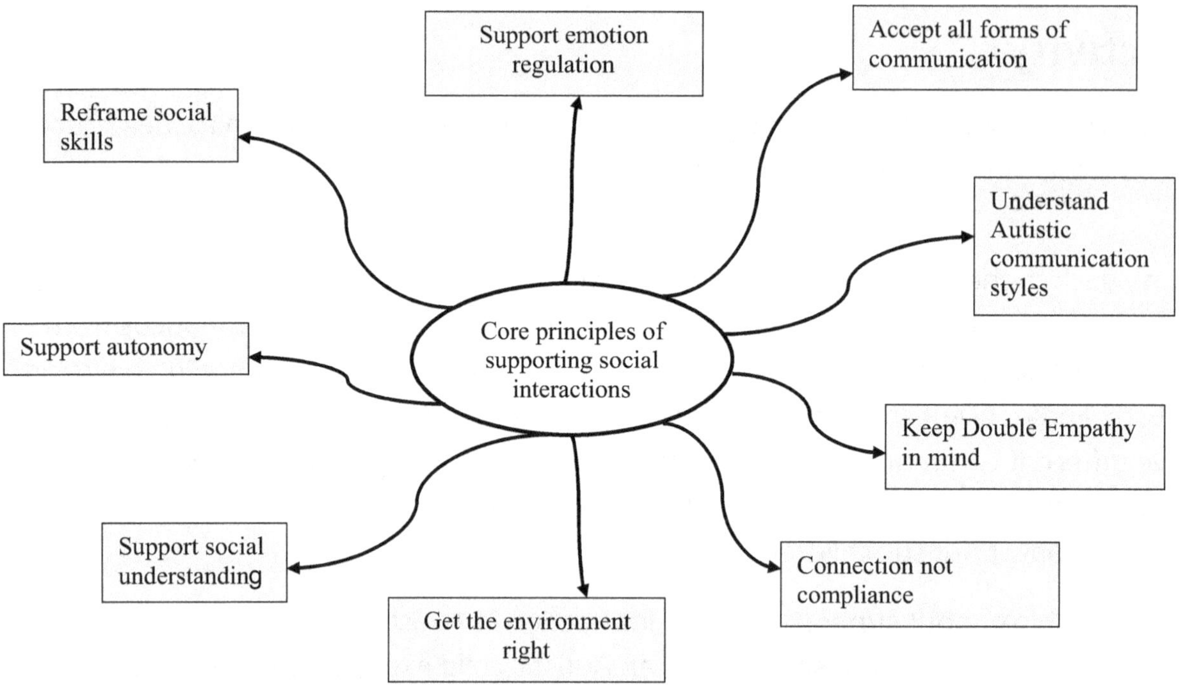

Figure 5.1 Core principles of supporting social interaction in Autistic children

Keep Double Empathy in mind:

- A key principle of Double Empathy is 'how to bridge the gap'. We need to think about what the world and interaction is like for an Autistic child. We can keep the core principles in mind to support this.
- For example, when we understand different communication styles, we accept all communication forms and don't seek to change things. Many of the conversations that I have in my work with Autistic children look different than conversations I have with neurotypical children.

Get the environment right:

- The physical and sensory environment has a huge impact on a child's ability to engage. We can all relate to this and recall times in busy, noisy and unpredictable environments where interaction and engagement feel harder. Similarly reflect on how much easier it is in a calm and predictable environment with 'someone who gets you'.
- Autistic children may prefer smaller groups with predictable routines. They may prefer side by side interactions and find large groups overwhelming.

Connection not compliance:

- This means that the priority should be a child's level of connection, sense of safety and trust in communication partners. This is more important than a child sitting still, following instructions and appearing 'well behaved'.
- When adults get too focussed on the wrong things (e.g. eye contact and sitting still) this can lead to a child feeling misunderstood and pressured, or worse unsafe. This can lead to masking, anxiety and meltdowns and shutdowns.
- When we prioritise connection, we support children to engage joyfully in a way that makes sense for them.

Support social understanding:

- Many of the older primary and secondary aged children often come to sessions with questions around social understanding. This often entails them asking me about the social behaviours of others so we can problem solve them together, for example why someone may act a certain way or say something. I often think of supporting social understanding as helping a child to navigate; as with any good journey the child needs to be motivated by the destination. With this in mind we can support social understanding and social problem solving in situations that the child is motivated by to help the world make sense. A good example of this is supporting a child to understand the intentions of others that they may otherwise find overwhelming and confusing.

Support autonomy:

- It is important that children are able to say 'no' and not have to engage in social situations when they don't want to or are overwhelmed. This is the start of 'self-advocacy' and starting early is important to hear the child's voice and not put pressure on them to mask.

Reframe social skills:

- We don't need to teach Autistic children to act like neurotypical children. Instead, we are supporting connection and authentic communication whilst helping a child to build tools that are useful to them.

I worked with Flora who loves Pokémon; her older siblings trade Pokémon cards and play Pokémon games with their friends. She is really motivated to join in but finds it hard to use language to join in. She was really motivated to learn social phrases that enabled her to join in.

Support emotion regulation:

- We can all relate to this one. When we are calm and ready, in 'just the right state', interaction is always going to be easier than when we are anxious.
- Within the early years environment, we can support emotion regulation by tuning into a child's likes and dislikes, through close communication with parents around whether the child has slept/eaten well, etc.

Understand Autistic communication styles:

- In Chapter 4 we discussed that an Autistic communication style might look different from what we see in neurotypical children. Understanding that this is a difference and not a deficit is a key principle to keep in mind. There may be differences in an Autistic child's verbal and non-verbal communication, for example less eye contact, a preference for parallel play, echolalia, differences in using and understanding tone and facial expressions. Differences in conversation may include 'info dumping' and less 'small talk' or favouring certain topics and talking about them lots of times. None of these are deficits. Autistic children under five may not like 'chit chat'. I met a little boy recently who illustrated this. His mum and nursery had raised some concerns that he didn't always respond and tended to always want to talk about his own things. On the way to the clinic room, I asked his mum about the journey and his snack; he changed the topic and talked about trains.
- Often younger Autistic children can find it hard to know the 'entry point' to a conversation. This means that they may begin talking animatedly mid topic. A child may find it hard to start an interaction verbally and may do this physically. This is not them 'butting in' or interrupting.
- An Autistic child may need more processing time and will benefit from a clear and direct communication style where adults mean what they say and say what they mean. They will benefit from adults 'waiting' as they process longer instructions.
- An Autistic child may choose a preferred topic to connect; recognising a child's special interest is important.

- Recognising and understanding Autistic communication styles help to build skills without putting pressure on a child, which can cause increasing masking and compliance.

Tip

Things to avoid: asking a child to look at you, saying 'use your words', forcing social behaviours and conventions that make a child feel uncomfortable or distressed.

I met Finn in nursery recently. The key worker asked, 'can you play with Leo?' Finn responded 'yes', but continued playing with the trains. The key worker expressed some frustration that Finn had not listened. I expressed that Finn was merely responding literally, in his mind possibly thinking 'yes I can play with Leo' but not gauging that this question meant 'go and play with Leo now'. We discussed reframing the language used and thought about what the key worker needed to include in the statement to tell Finn that firstly trains were finished and secondly to give him a choice of who to engage with and what activity to select. Statements like 'go and play' are very abstract for a child to understand; using clear and direct language such as first bikes, then play dough is always going to be clearer.

Often, I have visited nurseries and asked who or what a child likes to play with to be met with a response, 'He's really happy on his own. He likes to do his own thing'. Whilst this may appear to be the case, we have a key role in making social interaction accessible as well as motivating and fun for Autistic children so that they are able to participate if this is something motivating to them. Being able to help children make connections and have a shared social focus can be really powerful and impactful for them and their families.

I am often astounded at the small tweaks we need to make to our interaction to have a huge impact on a child. In my work with parents, I often have them doing all sorts of silly things that their child finds motivating. I will always remember working with a dad who found it difficult to know how to engage with his child, which led to the dad feeling overwhelmed and unsure where to start. His child knew colours and numbers and loved matching games but Dad and him found connecting in activities difficult. Within a few weeks the father was crawling around the floor like a horse, playing chasing games and a game they had invented jumping on a cushion; his child was showing shared enjoyment, connection and joy with lots of laughing and requesting the interaction to continue. It was such a pleasure to observe and facilitate. Therapy approaches that seek to support parents in connecting with their children are helpful for children under five. You may have heard of the following programmes which are run by SLTs. The PACT programme (Green et al., 2010), which is a parent-mediated social communication intervention designed to improve interaction between caregivers and Autistic children, and More Than Words® (Sussman, 2012), which focuses on coaching parents to support social communication in everyday routines.

This chapter looks in more detail at social interaction and provides practical ideas and strategies to support this. The areas that have been covered in previous chapters are closely related; communication and interaction go hand in hand and are strongly impacted by the environment.

Many early education environments and nurseries for children under five years are structured around neurotypical norms. This leaves young Autistic children to adapt to systems that were not designed with their needs in mind. The following case studies highlight how misunderstanding can often arise in relation to social interaction.

Lana is Autistic; she is three years old. She has been at nursery for one year and has settled in well to the routine. She has a good relationship with her key worker and enjoys chasing games and songs which she will now initiate. She loves messy play activities, and staff are expanding her range of play using her interests. When Lana is excited, she flaps her hands and vocalises. Lana does not use words consistently to communicate but staff are tuned into her, so they are often able to anticipate her needs. A theatre group is coming to nursery and has planned a group activity during which the children need to make a mask. When the group arrives, Lana is unable to sit and take part and walks away from the group. Later on, she is excited by the adults singing and waving scarves and joins in, running around and vocalising. The adult running the group has limited understanding of Autism and thinks Lana is badly behaved and rude.

It's important to prepare for out of routine activities. It is also helpful for staff to let visitors know that Lana is Autistic and communicates and engages in a different way from the other children. This means that they can consider changing the activity or bringing something for Lana. When unfamiliar people are visiting your setting, let them know that you have an Autistic child. You could signpost them to the National Autistic Society website (www.autism.org.uk).

Seren is four and a half; he has a detailed and rich knowledge and vocabulary relating to transport and planets. He loves talking about these and talking about them makes him feel secure and safe as well as bringing him joy. He sometimes talks more about his strong interests if he is unsure and anxious about what is happening. On a recent trip to the farm with nursery, Seren talks at length with a parent volunteer about the machinery on the farm. The volunteer knows that he is different from the other children but finds it hard to find a way to engage with him. The volunteer feels ill equipped to know how to respond.

Seren needs to be prepared for the farm trip; it is not fair on him to be with an unfamiliar communication partner in an out of routine situation. Consider sharing a communication profile with new people.

Freddie is four years old. He has just been diagnosed as Autistic, and the much older paediatrician has mentioned that he is very high functioning. Parents were a little bit confused by this and haven't yet shared the diagnosis with everyone as it feels too overwhelming; there's a lot to read and process. Freddie tends to mask his differences and holds it together in situations until he is back in a safe place. Lots of people around him do not notice his differences. Freddie likes his peers and works hard to engage in conversations. Freddie is an anxious boy as he is masking and working hard at all times. He also has some differences in his non-verbal communication where he tends to show the same facial expression and tone of voice. His face rarely changes even when he is excited or sad, which means that other people around him can rarely tell if he is feeling anxious or overwhelmed. He recently went to a birthday party of a friend – one of the parents commented to Freddie's mum that he seemed a bit miserable and looked like he wasn't having a nice time as 'he didn't look very happy'.

Ahmed is Autistic; he is three and a half years old. Ahmed loves to hug people and will hold children at nursery tightly. He recently tried to hug a stranger on the bus, which caused his mum concern. The stranger has an Autistic nephew and understood; he responded with kindness.

Rosa is four; she doesn't have an Autism diagnosis but has been referred for assessment. Her difficulties are subtle as she appears on the surface to join in; however, staff have increasingly noticed that often she will mimic what the other girls say. She has one particular friend, and if this child is not present, Rosa can appear a little lost. Rosa clearly wants to engage but at times seems unsure what to do. Rosa seems worried and anxious and picks her fingers and scratches the skin on her arms. Staff don't think that she is Autistic but are worried about her level of anxiety.

It is important to see the child holistically and understand that communication and social interaction difficulties can cause significant anxiety. Try not to separate out different observations, instead step back and consider how they may be linked.

Supporting social interaction in the early years

In the early years there is much that can be done to support interaction in Autistic children. Through changing the environment and not the child we can provide:

- Social opportunities
- Positive social experiences
- Opportunities for shared enjoyment with peers

Even though 'social interaction' is a separate chapter, it is very much linked to the previous chapters. The strategies outlined in Chapters 3 and 4 also support interaction. It makes sense that if the environment is right, and you can communicate your needs and preferences, it becomes easier to engage.

In Chapter 4 we talked about joint and shared attention and how we could establish these (C:1) using motivating activities and also imitation (C:3). Making a connection with a child is of key importance to developing early communication and interaction skills.

Tips for making a connection

- Consider what the children are interested in and join them in their activity rather than imposing your own.
- Imitate (C3).
- Be playful and engage in fun, motivating games.
- Don't be self-conscious; the children you are working with will appreciate you getting down to their level and putting in the effort to connect with them.

- Get down to a child's level. This sounds like such a simple tip, but it makes all the difference. You may need to lie down on your front – whatever you need to ensure you are at the same level. This may be face to face or side by side. For some children face to face may feel too much.

Tips for educators to support social interaction

- Say what you mean and mean what you say – much of social interaction is reliant on non-verbal communication; this can at times be confusing for Autistic children. Where other children may pick up on more subtle social cues, such as changes in an adults' facial expressions or tone of voice, an Autistic child may need you to tell them clearly what is expected. The example that always comes to mind is when a teacher stands with finger on lips making a 'shhhh' gesture – neurotypical children are able to tune in and understand that this means all be quiet now. An Autistic child may need the adult to give context to this, to get down to their level and show them on the first/next board what is happening next and to give an idea of what to do.
- Give clear language to accompany your facial expressions; this will help children make the social connection. Emotions can be abstract for Autistic children to process. If you can act as a guide and provide extra information about what is happening at the time it is happening, this can be helpful; for example, 'Salma, you look really happy. I can see you are smiling. I think it is because you like playing with the dolls'.
- As mentioned, all of the communication strategies outlined in Chapter 4 are extremely relevant for supporting social interaction. Naturally most of the activities that you do are targeting both areas; for example, during pauses you may find that as well as using a word to request, a child may also have a moment of connection with you.
- Be predictable in your interactions; to start off play games the same way. This gives Autistic children time to figure out what they are expected to do. Once the game is established you can introduce new elements or start to teach flexibility as part of the routine.
- If it is a favourite game and the child really likes it there is nothing wrong with playing the same game again and again.
- Be realistic and give time to practise skills; for example, practise taking turns or a new game with an adult before expecting a child to do it in a small group with other children who may be more unpredictable.

- Pausing is a powerful tool. Pause as part of interactions and wait expectantly to give a child a cue to continue the game.

What not to do

- One common 'don't do' that sometimes happens is when adults demand Autistic children to look at them. We want communication and interaction to be spontaneously joyful rather than being demanding of a child.
- Don't try to impose your agenda on a child and make him or her conform to what everyone else is doing. We need to change ourselves and not the child. Through changing ourselves, using positive strategies and adapting our environment, we can have a positive impact on social communication and interaction skills.
- Try to avoid emotional demands for example, 'It will make me very happy if you sit still', or 'walking calmly makes teachers feel proud'; most Autistic children in the early years will struggle to understand this and it is very unlikely to be motivating to them.
- Don't take offence if a child doesn't respond to you in a typical way.

S:1 Social interaction activity sheet 1. A shared social experience

S:1

As early years educators you are in an ideal position to facilitate positive social experiences for Autistic children. Some Autistic children may have had limited opportunities with other children, and those that they may have had (in the park or at toddler groups) may not have involved a shared and joint focus and opportunities for connection. This may sound silly as in a nursery environment there are children everywhere! However, I often visit children in an early years setting to consistently see them playing with their own activity in the same corner of the nursery. Whilst there may be times when a child does just want and need to be alone, it is also important to provide opportunities for social connection with peers that are accessible and meaningful to an Autistic child. I have often been met with 'he can't do circle time', so the child is seldom included. Remember, 'change yourself, not the child'. Consider how you can adapt your circle time activity so that it is motivating for an Autistic child in your setting. One setting I visited did exactly this and decided to incorporate a parachute game at the end of every circle time. This worked really well in enabling the child to join in and have a positive shared social experience.

Involve and educate other children

Many years ago, I was lucky to work in a wonderful Autism resource base attached to a mainstream school. The teacher actively educated neurotypical children in the mainstream school around how best to interact and support Autistic children. This very much sits with the premise that we shouldn't only be teaching Autistic children to adapt; approaches that do this are missing the point that social interaction is a two-way process, and neurotypical children also need to learn how to communicate and interact inclusively. In this particular school, children from the mainstream were taught key principles of intensive interaction and had lots of opportunities to use this with their Autistic peers. This worked so well, and created wonderful opportunities for connection and shared enjoyment between peers. In fact, many of the Autistic children responded far better to other children than an adult educator. By including the peers of Autistic children we are supporting inclusive practice. Many children love having a role; being a helper and showing another child can be highly motivating.

When an Autistic child has a shared social experience, you may notice the following:

- Joining in the activity alongside other children
- Looking

- Smiling
- Shared enjoyment
- Joint and shared attention (C:1)

Remember, the aim is to provide an opportunity and activity where these can happen rather than having an expectation of what the interaction will look like.

Activity ideas for a shared social experience

- Tailoring to the individual child and their preferences
- Music and dancing – supports gestalt language processors
- Parachute games

Materials needed

- Tailored activities to the child's interests

S:2 Social interaction activity sheet 2. A shared social focus

S:2

Remember, social interaction starts with a shared social experience that is motivating. Shared attention and enjoyment are an important part of social interaction. Sometimes we can get bogged down in trying to develop skills that are simply too hard. So often I visit children in their nursery where there is an emphasis on taking turns and sharing; some children aren't ready for this, and there are other more meaningful skills to focus on before this.

To develop interaction, a shared social focus can be a good starting point. This overlaps with developing joint attention as outlined in (C:1).
A shared social focus needs to be motivating for the child and may involve the following:

- Focussing on the same activity, song or interactive sequence
- Smiling
- Laughing
- Shared attention and enjoyment

Once you have a shared social focus you can do the following:

- Give meaning to a child's actions
- Engage in two-way, reciprocal interaction

Throughout this manual we have emphasised the philosophy of 'change yourself, not the child' – you can adapt what you are doing in motivating interactions to give Autistic children a chance to engage.

To start off with, a child may not come and ask you to play or interact in a way that you are expecting. You can use the following strategies to create a social focus:

- Get to the child's level.
- Imitate a child's actions, sounds and movements (C:3).
- Be playful. Play beside them rather than being directive.
- Use their interests and preferences, e.g. if a child loves trains or Dora Explorer bring these.
- Tune into sensory preferences in play, e.g. water, sand.
- Understand a child's motivations in people games (games without toys), e.g. a song, tickling or chase me.
- Use pausing (C:2).

- Slow down – this can be one of the most powerful strategies. Typically, interaction happens so quickly and naturally. If we can slow down and repeat our actions, we create predictability and give processing time. This makes it easier to join in.
- Repeat, repeat, repeat; an Autistic child will benefit from the activity happening many times, so they become familiar with what is expected of them.

S:3 Social interaction activity sheet 3. Making a chance to interact

S:3

Once we have created a shared social focus, we can use strategies as part of motivating games and interactions to encourage a child to join in games that are interesting and motivating to them and to request more of favoured games and interactions.

The strategies and activities that you have learnt in Chapter 4 on communication are relevant to interaction. Rather than applying them to requesting objects, toys or snacks, they can be applied to interaction. Recap activity sheets (C:2), (C:5) and (C:7). We will look now at how we can apply the strategies of pausing, giving and using a ready, steady, go game as part of an activity.

To make a chance for a child to interact we need to do the following:

- Slow the interaction down and use the appropriate language level.
- Start the game the same way.
- Use consistent words, gestures and props.
- Incorporate pauses.
- Finish the game the same way.

Peekaboo

- **Start the game the same way** – Show the scarf and put it on your head.
- **Use consistent words, gestures and props** – Sing, 'Where is (your name)?'
- **Incorporate pauses** – Pause (the child may pull down the scarf), then you say, 'Boo'.
- **Finish the game the same way** – Say, 'five, four, three, two, one, hiding has finished' and put the scarf away.

As the children become familiar with the game, they may request more of the activity by giving (C:5), for example, giving you the scarf to put on your head. When we pause (C:2), we give them a chance to do this.

Ready, steady, go

We talked about ready, steady, go games in (C:7). This strategy lends itself nicely to tickling games or chasing games (and many more). Use your knowledge of a child to think about how you can incorporate this strategy.

- Start the game; for example, say 'Tickle', show a gesture and then tickle toes.
- Use facial expressions and tone to create interest and excitement.

- Say, 'Ready, steady', wait with your hands poised to tickle, and then say, 'Go'.
- Pause and wait expectantly to see what happens.
- Children may say 'Go' or grab your hands or look at you to show that they want the tickling to continue.
- Remember to wait expectantly and excitedly. To start off, you may need to wait for at least five to ten seconds.
- Respond to any attempt to communicate made by the child, for example, looking, reaching or making a sound.

S:4 Social interaction activity sheet 4. Making interaction predictable by adding structure

S:4

Social interactions can be unpredictable, which means that Autistic children can find it difficult to know what the expectations are; it can be hard for a child to know when they are supposed to take a turn and what that turn looks like. By focussing on practical social games and routines, we can bring predictability to interactions to support children with their ability to take part consistently. We have discussed how important structure is to Autistic children. By bringing structure to interactions, we make it easier. Conscious and deliberate planning can make activities more structured.

You can use the activity planner in Table 5.2 to help structure interaction. This can be printed and kept as a record which supports adult communication partners in being consistent. See Table 5.3 as a completed example.

Table 5.2 Let's interact: planning sheet

Let's interact: planning sheet!	
Child's name: Date:	
Activity: Think about what is fun/ motivating, e.g. chase me, peek a boo, favourite song. Or a more structured playground game, e.g. What's the time Mr. Wolf	
What is the aim? Personalise for each child, for example: - to take a turn in a play routine - to create a social connection - to communicate a preference in a game	
Materials needed: (materials for the activity and also support, e.g. core boards, choosing boards)	
Strategies I will use (myself and environmental):	
How will I start the activity?	
How will I finish the activity?	
Activity observations: think about what went well – would you do anything differently next time?	
Observations: (child) include language sample	

Table 5.3 Let's interact: completed planning sheet example

Let's interact: planning Sheet!	
Child's name: Rosa Date: 16.9.2026	
Activity: Think about what is fun/ motivating, e.g. chase me, peek a boo, favourite song. Or a more structured playground game, e.g. What's the time Mr. Wolf	What's the time Mr Wolf at breaktime, Rosa really wants to be involved with her peers but is unsure how to
What is the aim? Personalise for each child for example: - to take a turn in a play routine - to create a social connection - to communicate a preference in a game	To provide a structured interaction and positive social experience for Rosa to join her peers in
Materials needed: (materials for the activity and also support, e.g. core boards, choosing boards).	How to play What's the time Mr Wolf script? Adults to read this to Rosa
Strategies I will use: (myself and environmental)	Choose a quieter part of the playground Let Rosa choose who is going to be the wolf; choosing the game is too much of an overwhelming choice but allowing choice within the game is helpful. Model social language Offer autonomy and self-advocacy as soon as Rosa wants to finish the game; this should be respected
How will I start the activity?	Offer Rosa a choice to be involved. Use tape on the floor to make a line where to stand to start and a spot for where the wolf can go.
How will I finish the activity?	Agree with Rosa, does the game finish after everyone has had a turn being the wolf? Or when the bell rings? Remember to talk her through what happens if it is in the middle of her turn when the bell rings.
Activity observations: think about what went well – would you do anything differently next time?	Rosa responded really well to having read the script as she was aware of what the rules were. Problem solving also really helped as the bell rang mid Charlotte's turn, and Rosa said, 'we can play again next time'.
Observations: (child) include language sample	Rosa used the following language: 'Again, can I be the wolf?' 'Come on Charlotte' 'I love this game'

S:5 Social interaction activity sheet 5. Adding social language

In (C:12) we talked about adding language. As well as adding descriptive language and action words to enrich a child's language, we can also add and model social language around preferences and connection. Modelling the right language to a child during interaction is a positive way to develop social phrases that are useful for them. For GLP language learners we need to model declarative language that will be helpful to a child in social interaction.

We need to think about the language that the child needs. What language is going to be helpful to them? When we listen to children, they often share joy and connection over funny and silly words, and it is just as important, if not more important, to be modelling these than what would be thought of as more conventional social language. I often come across targets for children where a child needs to greet a peer. When I observe children, I don't often see them saying 'hello Alex', they tend to say the name and go and play together. Modelling names is a really important part of making social language meaningful for a child. I remember being at a mud kitchen in the playground with an Autistic child and peers and I was modelling 'stinky mud', 'that's yucky' and 'that stinks'; this created a really age-appropriate moment of shared joy and connection as all the other three-year-olds found this really funny.

We need to model social language that helps Autistic children with a range of functions, as summarised in Table 5.4. It is important to tune into this instead of just teaching 'say hello' or 'say sorry' or 'ask for a turn'.

Remember to model social language in the moment.

Table 5.4 Examples of useful and functional social language

Function		*Examples*
Connect	⟷	These can help with the entry point to interaction, e.g. 'can I play?', 'Let's play', 'watch this', 'look', 'my turn', 'your turn'. Knowing peers' names is also helpful to support connection as well as words like 'wow', 'that's silly'!
Express preferences and have boundaries	⟷	This can help with self-advocacy, e.g. 'No', 'stop', 'I need space', 'leave me', 'I want to play alone', 'I need a break'.
Flexibility and negotiation	⟷	These are really important skills that are often overlooked in peer interactions, e.g. 'after this', 'next turn', 'maybe later', 'you choose'.
Repair when things go wrong	⟷	This can help with managing misunderstandings which are a normal part of interaction, e.g. 'stop', 'help', 'that's mine', 'can I have it back?', 'let's try again', 'shall we do something different?'.
Join in, in a way that feels safe	⟷	This can help with expressing feelings in play, e.g. 'I'm happy', 'I feel sad', 'I don't like that', 'too loud', 'that's funny!', 'I'm excited!'

S:6 Social interaction activity sheet 6. Taking turns

S:6

Turn taking is often an area of focus for Autistic children. Turn taking can be difficult for all children. Often, we try to get children to take turns in activities that are too difficult for them, for example, a game with another child or handing over a toy. Taking turns and sharing actually involves numerous, quite complex thought processes which can be difficult for lots of children. Being able to take turns in a specific game involves children being able to wait. Recap (E:6) as this may be a useful cue to include when you are encouraging children to take turns. We can rethink turn taking as it doesn't have to be within a game with waiting, it can be part of natural, low-pressure interactions, such as sharing ideas, exchanging sounds, taking turns adding pieces to a construction, commenting on a shared interest or engaging in back-and-forth play. This approach allows children to experience the rhythm of interaction in a way that feels meaningful, enjoyable and less demanding.

Top tips for taking turns

- Vocal turn taking with an adult can be a great place to start and relates to (C:2). When a child makes a sound, copy him or her. This non-pressured play activity is an easy way to take turns.
- Turn taking can be as simple as rolling a ball to each other or rolling a car down a ramp. Keep the turns quick and fun and in line with a child's interests.
- If turn taking in a more structured game with peers, it can be helpful to practice with an adult first. This gives lots of positive social opportunities and time for modelling language.
- Use consistent language, for example, 'My turn'. You may introduce waiting as well as other visual supports such as a first/next board as a child becomes more familiar with the concept of taking turns. Use a gesture to indicate whose turn it is.
- Use quick games to start with. If a turn is taking too long and the child needs to wait too long, you can lose the focus of turn taking, and it becomes more about waiting. Quick turns allow a child to become involved quickly.
- Use a child's interests and motivations to keep it fun.
- Use predictable activities in which the turns are fairly consistent.
- Once a child is familiar with a turn-taking game, bring in other children.
- If you are using a prop or game as part of the interaction, make sure that it isn't too motivating for the child to just want to take the object and focus on it themselves.

Games for quick turn taking

- Roll a ball
- Bubbles for...
- Hiding (peekaboo with a scarf) – this also provides an opportunity for giving and for the child to initiate the game
- Cause-and-effect pop-up type toys
- Bricks for making a tower where you each take a turn

Materials needed

- None for vocal turn taking and imitation
- Games for quick turn taking

S:7 Social interaction activity sheet 7. Taking turns – making it visual

S:7

Turn taking is quite complicated! Before starting with turn-taking games, it is important to build social connection and positive social opportunities for a child! What is the point in being able to take turns if you haven't had a chance to connect and share joy?

When, and only when, a child is ready to join in more structured turn-taking games, we need to consider how we present the activities to increase structure so that they are more predictable.

I often hear comments like 'he's not good at sharing', 'she can't take turns' in activities that are really abstract. We need to consider how we add visual supports and clear structure that can make the game more predictable to support participation. It is also really important alongside turn taking to continue to model lots of social language (C:5).

By adding structure to turn taking, we can help children understand

- Whose turn it is
- How long the turn is going to be

What structure can we add?

- Wait card
- Turn-taking board (S:8)
- Use of sand timers/countdown timers
- Use of a script or social story

Activity

Think about an existing activity that you regularly use in your setting. How can you bring more structure to support Autistic children to take turns as part of the activity?

Outside equipment

I once worked with a specialist nursery where we set a great system to support turn taking for their outside play equipment. They put the following in place:

- A photo board with pictures of all of the equipment, including bikes, push carts and so on.
- Photographs of the children were used to support understanding of the sequence of turns. Everyone had a choice of what they wanted and this was presented clearly and visually.
- Use of two-minute sand timers indicated how long each turn was. Staff used a five, four, three, two, one countdown and the children were all really clear around when to swap and take turns.
- Staff consistently carried wait cards on their lanyards to offer a visual cue.
- There was consistent use of social language around 'my turn', 'waiting' and 'finished' as well as language to share joy and connection.

S:8 Social interaction activity sheet 8. Using a turn-taking board

S:8

This visual is helpful to use for children as part of a more structured game with quick turns for children who understand 'wait'. Using of a wait card alongside the board would be helpful. Children need to know a little bit about turn taking before introducing this, otherwise it will feel frustrating for them.

Instructions for turn-taking board

- Copy the board (Figure 5.2).
- Colour in the borders of the top frame so it is green and cut it out before laminating so that it is clear in the middle.
- Colour in the borders of the four bottom squares so they are red.
- Laminate.
- Write the names or place a photo of who is in the group in a red square.
- Indicate whose turn it is by placing the green square over the top.

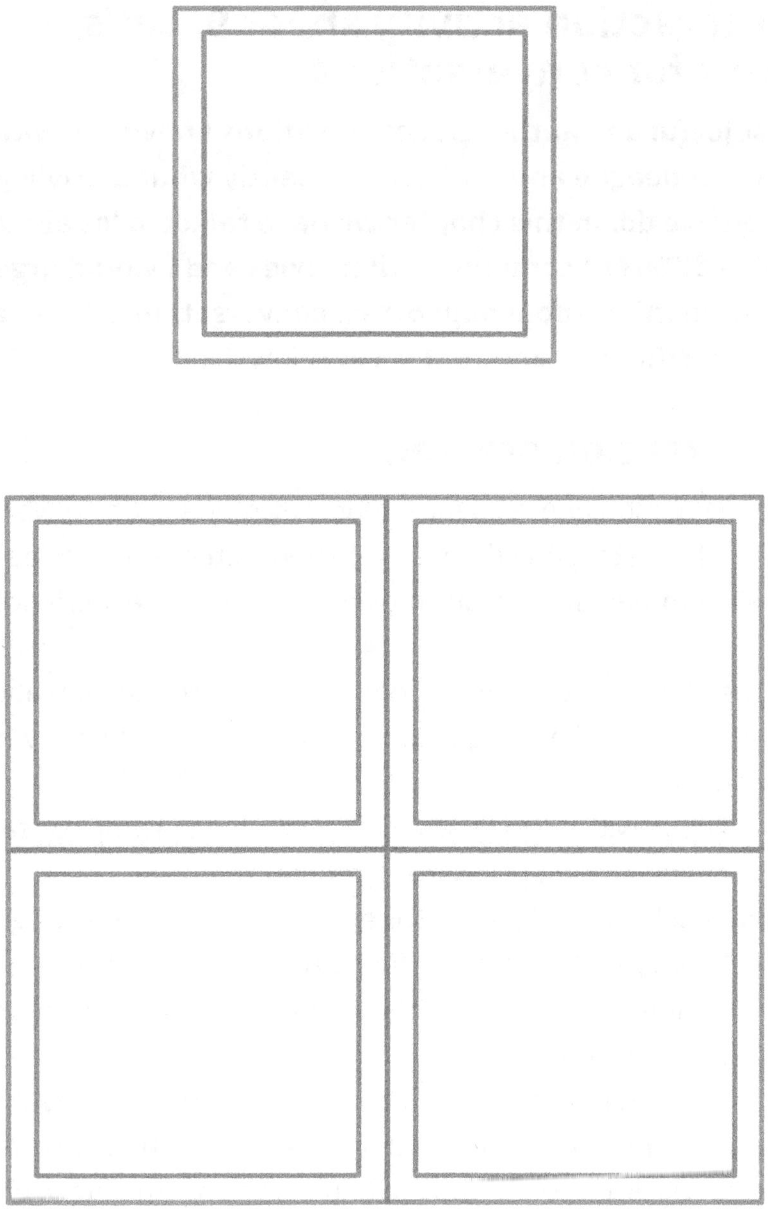

Figure 5.2

S:9 Social interaction activity sheet 9. Let's chat – top tips for conversations

S:9

Some of the most joyful and authentic conversations I have are with Autistic children. A colleague and I reflected recently what a privilege it is to be able to do the work we do. In this chapter we have talked a lot about respecting and understanding different communication styles and I would urge you to hold this in mind when we think about supporting conversations. A recognition that conversation will be different, and that is ok, is key.

Get the conversation started

- Tune into a young person and recognise that they may start a conversation in their own way. Rather than expecting them to gain your attention first, look for and respond to their comments, interests, movements, shared experiences or bids for connection.
- Reduce your questions; instead, make comments. Often a conversation can feel like an interview with more and more questions being asked of a child which can lead to them shutting down.
- Model social language with no pressure to repeat, don't prompt or say, 'say...'
- Model social language with no pressure to repeat.
- Offer conversational leads and pause; for example, instead of saying 'What did you do over the weekend?', say, 'Something funny happened to me over the weekend'.
- Talk about a child's interests and allow time for this; learn about these as it will create an opportunity to connect.
- Do something wrong on purpose as a funny way to start a conversation; for example, try to pour the juice with the lid on or say something incorrectly. If you know a child is good with colours, you could try labelling one incorrectly; wait to see if he or she corrects you.
- Give a context for conversations, for example, looking at a book or magazine, or adding social language (S:5), such as 'I like it' or 'That is my favourite'.

Use practical activities

- We know that when we provide a context, it is easier for children with Autism to engage. This makes the conversation less abstract.
- Use the child's about-me book (C:16) as a context to start the conversation.
- Engage in a practical activity (C:15) as a basis for conversation.
- Include other children in a practical activity; take photos of it and talk about it afterwards.

Remember, you are the social guide

- Ensure that the experience is positive for an Autistic child. Remember to respect self-autonomy and make sure that a child has a way to say 'no', to leave the group or to say they don't like it.
- As the adult, facilitate the child and repair the conversation if and when needed.
- Help the child build success.

S:10 Social interaction activity sheet 10. Supporting perspective taking

S:10

Perspective taking can emerge differently and at different times for Autistic children. This means that an Autistic child might find it hard to understand the thoughts, feelings and intentions of others. This can impact their social experiences as they are constantly trying to navigate a world that feels hard to understand. Autistic children are often trying to navigate sharing toys, turn taking, group play and emotional reactions from peers, all of which can feel overwhelming. When we support perspective taking, we help Autistic children to:

- Understand more about other people's reactions
- Feel more secure in social situations
- Feel less confused and anxious

The aim is to reduce social stress. It is important to recognise that perspective taking is complex and often something I work with in older primary and secondary students. The following list provides some age-appropriate starting points to support Autistic children in early years:

- **Use clear and direct language** – avoid ambiguous and non-literal language. Say what you mean and mean what you say.
- **Make it specific** – Autistic children find it hard to infer unspoken rules. If we can make 'unspoken' and abstract rules clearer, we are supporting perspective taking. It is also important to provide explanation for this rather than just 'because I said so'.
- **Help scaffold perspective taking by providing explanation** – e.g. 'I think that Marni is feeling sad because...'.
- **Talk about thoughts** – make these more concrete by drawing them out with a thought bubble.
- **Talk about feelings** – make it clear why someone is feeling a particular way; for example, 'Oh, look, Sam is so happy', or 'She is really smiling because she likes that ice cream'. Put your child's feelings and your own into words; for example, 'I'm excited today, I am really looking forward to your school show'.
- **Label and give context to a child's emotions**
- **Use books** – to comment on the thoughts, feelings and experiences of others. We can relate these back to personal experiences.

- **Talk about other people** – e.g. if Grandma's birthday is coming up, talk about what Grandma likes and what might be a good present for her.
- **Remember Double Empathy** – in addition to supporting Autistic children with understanding perspectives we need to ensure that peers and adults understand Autistic perspectives.

Materials needed

- None

Chapter 5 summary

- The social world can feel overwhelming for many Autistic children. We need to support Autistic children with participation in interactions that they are motivated to join in.
- Social interaction looks different for Autistic children and this is something that should be celebrated. Differences are not deficits and we are NOT trying to teach social skills.
- In the early years we can offer opportunities for positive social interaction and facilitate success. This doesn't always have to be turn taking and sharing; social success will depend on the individual child – for one child this may mean engaging in conversation; for another it may involve connecting and sharing joy as part of a special interest.
- We need to dispel harmful and outdated myths around social interaction in Autistic children.
- The environment has a big impact on engagement.
- Sensory difficulties can impact a child's ability to engage.
- Joint and shared attention are important skills to develop.
- By setting up a predictable environment (Chapter 3) and through providing consistent and appropriate support around communication (Chapter 4), we offer a good starting point to develop interaction.

References

Green, J., Charman, T., McConachie, H., Aldred, C., Slonims, V., Howlin, P., Le Couteur, A., Leadbitter, K. and Pickles, A. 2010. Parent-mediated communication-focused treatment in children with autism (PACT): a randomised controlled trial, *The Lancet*, 375(9732), pp.2152–2160.

Sussman, F. 2012 *More Than Words: Helping Parents Promote Communication and Social Skills in Children with Autism Spectrum Disorder*. 2nd edn. Toronto: The Hanen Centre.

6

Autistic play

Chapter 6 provides the following:

- An overview of how we can support play as part of a neuro-affirming approach
- Case studies illustrating how play can look different in Autistic children
- Guiding principles around being a supportive partner in play
- Strategies to use in play

Shifting perspectives

Throughout this manual we have highlighted shifting perspectives around understanding differences in Autistic children. As with communication and social interaction, Autistic play can look different from what we see in neurotypical children. As SLTs we have very much shifted from the perspective of 'how can we make this play look more typical?' to understanding that Autistic play is important and doesn't need changing. We have touched previously on the idea that neurotypical milestones are not helpful for Autistic children. This is true in relation to communication, social interaction and play, as well as other areas of development. This perspective was clearly reflected in the parent stories in Chapter 2. When you think about it, it makes sense to not be comparing a child to milestones that were not designed for them.

For me, the biggest change of the second edition is in this chapter on play. In my own work I have always celebrated engagement and interaction with Autistic children and very much followed a child's lead in play. However, at times in my working life I have been conflicted as many approaches seek to change or teach different kinds of play. In addition to this, outdated perspectives and reliance on milestones for neurotypical children have led to unhelpful narratives around play in Autistic children; some of these

DOI: 10.4324/9781003627760-6

have persisted and can be really harmful to Autistic children. These perspectives can lead to interventions or targets that are looking to 'change' play in an Autistic child. We need to view play differently; in simple terms we need to view play as a vehicle for an Autistic child to explore the world and as a way for them to regulate and connect.

A neuro-affirming approach recognises and embraces differences in Autistic play and highlights that the differences are purposeful, valid and meaningful. Play can look very different in individual Autistic children as the following case studies illustrate. When reading the case studies reflect on the fact that there is not one way to play that is better than the other.

Kitt is three years old and has an amazing ability to notice small details. He is very motivated by visual contrasts and often gets very absorbed in watching the movement in trees or rain falling on the window and the pattern it leaves behind. He can stand watching these for ages and this appears to make him very happy. At nursery he loves the sand tray and putting the sand through the sieve, which he will do again and again. He loves it when his key worker joins him with her own sieve, also passing the sand through it from different heights. They watch the sand together in parallel and Kitt shows his enjoyment by smiling and leaning on her. He reaches towards the sand as it falls and vocalises to communicate that he wants more.

Eliza is five years old and loves playing imaginative games. She has a rich imaginative world and often has a very clear idea of how play should be. She loves acting out scenarios from her nursery and TV programmes that she has watched. Although she wants other children and adults to join in and will ask them to do so, she can find it difficult when they do not follow her idea in play. This can lead to her feeling frustrated, particularly when other children are involved who do not respond in a predictable way. Staff have noticed that Eliza responds well when adults join but do not attempt to change the play.

Toby is four years old and loves little toy figures. At nursery he often goes to the dolls house and collects all the people and carries them around with him. He is highly motivated by the people and likes to move them along shelves and different surfaces. Toby has a GLP learning style, and his play is accompanied by lots of vocalisations with rich intonation. Staff initially thought that he may like to set the people up in the dolls house but he is not interested in this. They realise from observing him that he is using echolalia to narrate his play.

Table 6.1 Principles of play in Autistic children

Principles of play	
Play helps regulation	Many Autistic children use play as a way to feel good and to regulate themselves. Play actions can help a child to feel more regulated by providing predictability, reducing anxiety and creating a safe feeling through something that is rewarding to the child. It is therefore important not to look to 'stop' a particular kind of play. Play may involve focussing intently on a particular object or topic, it may include repetitive actions or have a sensory component; this is all ok.
Play builds communication	Play provides a shared social experience which gives a context for communication. When adults join a child's play and follow their lead they create opportunities for connection, shared and joint attention and communication.
Play supports autonomy	We have talked about the importance of autonomy and self-advocacy for Autistic children. Play can give an Autistic child the opportunity to be themselves, to engage in something deeply motivating, to make choices and express who they are. These are powerful experiences to support autonomy.
Play provides opportunities for social connection	Play that is motivating for a child provides an opportunity for social connection. When the environment is flexible and communication partners are responsive, Autistic children can engage in ways that feel safe and authentic. Connecting through a shared and motivating activity is meaningful. Special interests provide a context to connect. Play offers opportunities to be in parallel and together as a way to connect.
Play develops problem solving	Play can provide a vehicle for a child to develop problem solving skills as there are opportunities to experiment and test ideas. There are opportunities to collaborate and figure things out together in a non-pressured way.

We turn now to consider the importance of play and key principles. These are summarised in Table 6.1. This is not an exhaustive list and in your work, you may come up with more perspectives and principles.

Tip

Print Table 6.1 and use it as a discussion point to talk about play with your colleagues. Consider what else you would add.

Through respecting differences in play, communication partners are able to build trust to support connection, reduce stress through allowing access to predictable actions, support self-advocacy by allowing a child agency over what they do in their leisure time and build trust through allowing time and space to focus on activities that are important to the individual.

Many of the strategies that we have already discussed in supporting communication and social interaction are also applicable to supporting play. The following is not an exhaustive list but provides an overview.

Strategies for supporting play in Autistic children

- Don't see play with special interests as a reward or something that can only be done at special times. We should not be withholding items that are meaningful to a child. Play is an important part of being regulated and feeling safe and secure.
- Allow time for uninterrupted play; this may be recharging and supportive to a child's overall wellbeing.
- Observe and don't direct. Try to leave your agenda behind. Sometimes this can feel really difficult, especially if you have prepared an activity for a child and they are not motivated by it.
- Play in parallel to start with and wait to see if a child wants you to join. Don't just launch in.
- Be at the child's level; this will naturally make it easier for you to observe their interests.
- Follow the child's lead in play and attune to their interests.
- Don't ask questions, instead make comments.
- When the time is right, try narrating play using phrases and language from the child's perspectives.
- Leave time for silences and pauses!
- Look for connection and respond to all communication forms, whether this is verbal or non-verbal.
- Incorporate movement into play.
- Incorporate music; this is really helpful and supportive for children with a GLP learning style.
- Support sensory needs and consider the impact of the environment. There may be times when play changes depending on what is happening in the environment. Remember you can be a detective and observe a child across contexts.
- Offer choices of activities to support self-advocacy and choice. Remember there should always be an option to opt out or say no!
- Structure the environment to create predictability. Ensure there is access to quieter areas as well.

Activity

Think about the Autistic children you work with. What do you notice about their play? What works well in supporting them? Is there anything you could do differently

This chapter is slightly different from the previous ones as specific activity sheets are not provided. This is largely because we are not trying to 'change' a child's play, and really there is no right or wrong way to do it. Instead use the guiding principles and strategies in the children you work with. Be creative and have fun. I have included some of my favourite play ideas next!

Activity

Create your own list of play activities and add to these over time.

Use of a tent or quiet calming area – A tent can offer a quiet space for an Autistic child. If you don't have one, be creative and make a calming area.

Glittery water bottle – Add water, glitter and food colouring to a clear, two-litre bottle. Add some strong tape round the lid to ensure that there are no spillages. This can provide a really nice visual experience.

Making snow – Use squirty, child-friendly bath foam; this tends to be less strongly scented and is not irritating to skin. Make a big ball and clap, watch the snow fall.

Messy play – Try corn flour with water. Add colours and glitter, or encourage a child to get involved by including a favourite toy; for example, walk a dinosaur through.

Coloured spaghetti – You can create different-coloured spaghetti. In my experience children love this, and it can be fun to explore, plus there is no need to worry if it ends up being eaten.

- Cook spaghetti as usual.
- In a sealable bag add vegetable oil and food colouring.
- Add the spaghetti to the bag and leave for 15 minutes.
- Rinse excess colour from the spaghetti in cold water.

Moon sand – If you aren't familiar with moon sand, it is a great texture to mould, sieve and drive things through. It is easy and quick to make.

- Mix eight cups of flour and one cup of baby oil.
- I have added different smells as this can be interesting for some children to explore.

Bubble wrap popping – Walking or rolling on bubble wrap can be highly motivating and a great way to explore new textures and sounds.

Tinfoil blanket – This is one of my top therapy materials – great because they are inexpensive and can instantly transfer an activity, for example, peekaboo, hiding or pouring lentils onto it.

Shaking and pouring – Dry rice (which can also be coloured easily with food colouring) and lentils. Both can be very motivating, both visually and to listen to dropping on a tray.

Playing with a torch – A torch can be so fun in creating visual contrasts, creating shadows and different colours.

Let's create activities – As described in (C:15)

Chapter 6 summary

- Autistic play looks different and that is ok. We do not need to change a child's play.
- Play is a vehicle to build connection, communication, problem solving, autonomy and regulation.
- We need to tune into the child to learn more about their play.

7

Making sense of behaviour

Chapter 7 provides the following:

- Understanding behaviour
- Being a detective
- Using the iceberg model to problem solve behaviours
- Getting the basics right
- Prevention and preparation
- Top tips for managing behaviour

You may ask why there is a chapter on behaviour in a book about communication

Good question!

In my work with Autistic children, I am often saddened by the number of failed school placements and difficulties Autistic children face in the education environment. Whilst for some children a mainstream school environment is not right, for many children it is the lack of appropriate support and understanding that causes an education placement to breakdown. However, in my experience 'behaviour' is often cited as a reason why things don't work. The statistics on school exclusion for Autistic children are high; the sad reality is that for many Autistic children they are unable to access the right support and the impact of this is significant. For many children education can feel like 'being a square peg in a round hole' where nothing ever quite fits. The impact of this is huge and it is not in any way surprising that a child may not feel regulated or have high levels of anxiety in an environment that is not set up for them. We all have a responsibility to understand and make sense of behaviour, as very often in early years behaviour is a form of communication and is usually telling us something.

DOI: 10.4324/9781003627760-7

Often when the word behaviour is used there is a tendency to jump to conclusions and think that we mean a negative or challenging behaviour. In fact, behaviour is something we all do and is observable. A behaviour is influenced by the context it occurs in; for example, climbing itself is not a negative behaviour in the playground, but this can become problematic if you are climbing on the bookcases in the nursery. Similarly, something like handwashing is a behaviour we all do several times a day, usually at set points like after the toilet and before eating. There is nothing problematic with this behaviour unless it starts to occur intensively at lots of different times in the day. A lot of behaviours which are deemed challenging, such as hitting, pushing, biting and shouting out, are all behaviours that we see in all children.

When we talk about behaviour in this chapter there is not an implication that a behaviour is negative. The connotations of behaviour often conjure up a child who is making a choice to 'be naughty' or to have a tantrum. In actual fact, what we may be seeing is a child not feeling safe and secure, a very anxious child or a child having a meltdown or shutdown. This is a manual primarily about communication, so we don't discuss all of these ideas in huge detail; however, I would encourage you to read more about anxiety in Autism and the difference between tantrums and meltdowns and shutdowns as a good starting point.

I have learnt a lot from the wonderful clinical psychologists I have worked with who have taught me that rather than jumping in and looking immediately for a solution to a problem, we need to delve deeper and attempt to understand why the behaviour is occurring in the first place. Without this understanding, we will never reach the reason for the behaviour.

Making sense of behaviour – be a detective

We talked about the iceberg model in Chapter 2. This is really helpful in thinking about what is going on for a child under the waterline. The iceberg helps us to gather more information and problem solve 'why' a specific behaviour may be happening. Without this understanding it is difficult to come up with effective strategies. It is important to acknowledge that most of the iceberg is hidden under the water, and we see only the tip. This part is the behaviour. The majority is hidden under the water, and this is the reason as to why it is happening. When we just look at the tip of the iceberg, we fail to see what is going on underneath.

Take time to understand the 'why'. Talk to parents; get their thoughts. Gather information, *be a detective*. All too often we are keen to rush in and try different strategies before fully understanding the broader factors impacting a situation. The time you spend gathering information to see what is going on under the waterline is invaluable and will contribute to a far greater understanding of the issues and why they are happening, which ultimately leads you to a more effective solution. It can also be really helpful to think about the times when things are going well and what are the factors contributing to this.

The following case study about Jack and Ahmed highlights the importance in gathering the correct information so that you can really understand *why* a particular behaviour may be occurring. Without the 'why', it is difficult to put in place an effective strategy.

Behaviour observed: hitting

Jack and Ahmed attend the same early years setting. They are both Autistic and are often observed to be hitting different children. Staff have decided as a group to be consistent, say 'No hitting', and remove Jack or Ahmed from the situation when they hit. Unfortunately, the strategy isn't working for either child, and both children continue to hit other children. The behaviours are escalating, and other parents are commenting on both Jack and Ahmed hitting their children. This is also highly stressful for both sets of parents as well as for Jack and Ahmed.

On the advice of an SLT, staff decided to use the iceberg model as a way to gather more information about the behaviour.

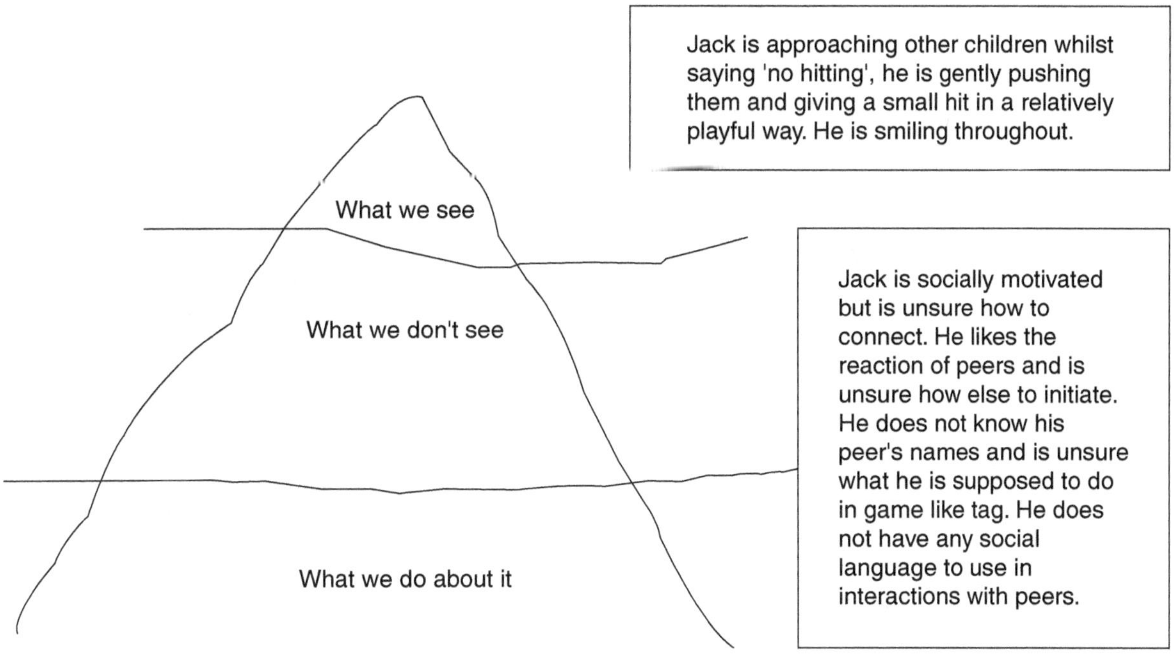

Figure 7.1 Jack's iceberg

From their observations they were able to conclude that Jack was using his behaviour as a way to communicate and interact with others.

What happened next?

- Staff working with Jack focussed on teaching him other ways to engage with peers.
- Instead of just saying 'No hitting', they focussed on teaching him alternative behaviours to replace the hitting. They modelled useful and helpful social phrases such as 'Can I play?', 'Chase me' and 'My turn'.
- Staff focussed on lots of structured paired activities with Jack which he loved.
- Staff also included Jack in a small social group with a focus on providing a positive shared social experience, turn taking and social language.

Ahmed found it difficult to cope at transition times. He found unstructured times between activities stressful. Ahmed is easily overwhelmed by the environment and wants to leave the situation. He has no way to tell anyone this. Using his behaviour to communicate is a quick and successful way to get himself out of a stressful situation.

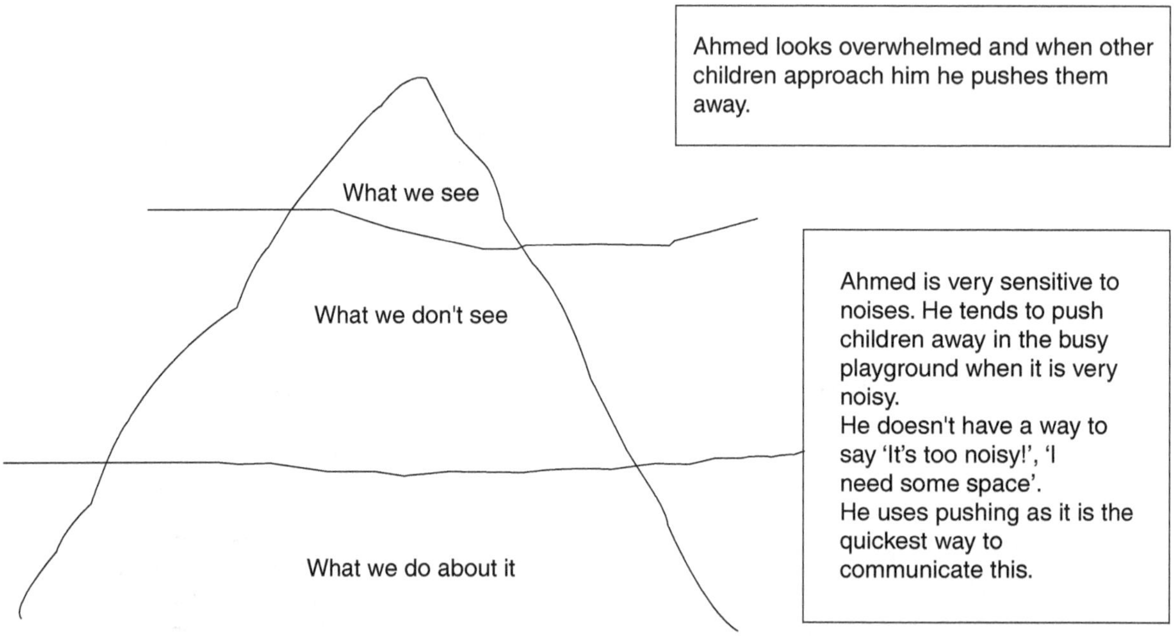

Figure 7.2 Ahmed's iceberg

What happened next?

- Staff working with Ahmed focussed on giving him a clear way to communicate 'no' or that he wanted to leave a situation; they effectively replaced the hitting behaviour with a communicative behaviour.
- Staff also helped reduce Ahmed's anxiety around transitions by increasing structure and using a portable visual timetable and first/next board; they also timetabled in more 'quiet time'.
- Collectively, these strategies saw an elimination of the hitting behaviours.

Jemima is Autistic and is four and a half years old. She is chatty and loves talking about Paw Patrol. Staff working with her report that she copes well in the early years environment. Occasionally she has a meltdown where she becomes very distressed; it takes her time to recover from this and it is upsetting for her. Staff can't understand why this happens. Jemima is unable to explain it. Staff working with Jemima do some detective work and discover that the meltdowns occurred when there were cut flowers in the reception area of the nursery. Staff talk to Jemima's mum, and she explained that Jemima is extremely sensitive to the smell of certain flowers. This case study highlights the impact that sensory factors can have on Autistic children. (I remember once talking to an Autistic adult who explained that the sound of wiping kitchen surfaces felt like it was 'cutting his ears'.)

Leon is three years and ten months. He is Autistic and has a few words that he uses to label colours and numbers. He has responded well to support from staff working with him focussing on copying his vocalisations and developing interactive games. Leon has recently started to bite staff hard on the shoulder. Staff feel that the behaviour comes from nowhere, and Leon often laughs when he is doing it. Staff want to know more about where the behaviour is coming from and how they can support Leon with what he is trying to communicate.

Staff do some detective work with the iceberg and keep a log of when this happens; they start to notice a pattern of when Leon would bite. It always tended to be after an enjoyable activity when he was excited. The adults' immediate response of a 'cross face and change of voice' was quite motivating for Leon and caused Leon to laugh. The adult responses seemed to be reinforcing the biting; essentially, he enjoyed what happened as a consequence to his biting and continued to do it.

What happened next?

- Staff met with Leon's parents to see if biting was happening at home.
- Staff agreed to all respond in a consistent yet neutral way, saying 'stop' in a calm voice and moving Leon away and onto a different activity with a neutral facial expression.
- Alongside this they focussed on modelling social language, e.g. 'I am excited' when Leon appeared excited. Staff also made sure that they were standing up when Leon started to get excited; this meant that they were naturally not in a place where he could bite them. Staff also made time for positive interaction and connection, using songs and people games so that Leon could share his excitement and joy at other times.
- Leon was also referred to OT as there seemed to be a sensory component to his biting (he also mouthed a lot of other toys).
- As a result, over a period of eight weeks, the biting reduced.

This example highlights that behaviour doesn't change quickly. Consistency is key in managing behaviour, and it's important to stick with strategies before feeling that they aren't working.

What's the trigger?

This is a question that I am often asked. Whilst sometimes there are clear triggers for behaviours, sometimes there are not. In many cases keeping a log around when a behaviour occurs and what happens before and after this can give us more clues about the situation; in many cases it doesn't. Conversely it can be helpful to keep a log of the times when a behaviour does not occur and the circumstances around this. It is important to acknowledge that for many Autistic children anxiety and stress increase throughout the day. This cumulative impact means that something seemingly small may happen and a child responds. If we just look at what happens immediately beforehand, we fail to take into account the broader situation. Even with supportive educators and good strategies in place, the early years environment can still be stressful and unpredictable which can cause increased stress and anxiety.

Recognising that there may not always be a clear trigger is helpful and important in acknowledging how difficult it can be for some children, especially if they are holding it together all day.

Activity

Think of an Autistic child who you work with or have worked with in the past. Were there ever behaviours that you were unsure as to why they occurred? Draw out an iceberg and be a detective to try and think more about how they occurred.

Preparation, prevention and getting the basics right

Essentially, we want to create an environment that is supportive in preventing behaviours from occurring. This does not mean that we are 'demanding compliance'; it means that we are tuning into a child and thinking about what they need to help them feel good in the environment. As a first step we need to get the basics right:

- This means having good communication with home. Ensuring that there is a nursery/schoolbook with key information included is important. This may be letting the setting know that a child has not had a good sleep or any other change in circumstances. I visited a child in nursery recently and the staff were discussing that his hitting had escalated; one of the staff causally remarked that it was probably because his mum was away with work. No one else was aware and the impact on his behaviour had not been considered.
- Sleep, eating, general wellbeing. All of these factors can impact any child's behaviour.
- Consistency and predictability are important; changes to the routine are important to be aware of so that a child can be supported. Prepare a child for out of routine events that may be stressful.
- Listen to parents, recognise that a child may 'hold it together all day'.
- Change the environment not the child. Consider what is happening in the sensory environment.
- Use the energy accounting framework to think about what 'deposits' and 'withdrawals' are happening in the day.

Energy accounting (Toudal and Attwood, 2024)

The energy accounting framework is a way of understanding how Autistic children use and manage their mental, emotional and sensory energy throughout the day. You might have heard of someone's 'social battery' or 'spoons theory', which are similar in terms of core principles.

Essentially energy accounting works on the idea that every activity in the day, including social interaction, sensory processing, transitions or communication, has an 'energy cost'. These can be either withdrawals (things that drain energy) or deposits (things that build energy back up) in the energy accounting system. Autistic children often expend significantly more energy on everyday tasks that other children may find effortless. For example, coping with noise in a classroom, interpreting social cues or switching between activities can quickly drain their available energy. When energy runs low there are reduced reserves to manage daily demands. Therefore, they may need more time to deposit energy through engaging with a preferred activity or having access to breaks to recharge them. In my work with older children and teens this is an incredibly helpful framework to use, and we often talk about the withdrawals and deposits across the day and how they can be balanced to ensure that withdrawals don't exceed deposits.

In early years, educators can use this framework in a helpful way to:

- Recognise signs of fatigue or overload before a child becomes distressed
- Balance high-energy and high-demand activities with rest and low-demand activities
- Adjust expectations and the environment to reduce unnecessary energy expenditure
- Support self-regulation by allowing breaks, predictability and recovery time

In early years, this approach is especially helpful because young Autistic children can't often communicate when they are feeling overwhelmed. By making sure withdrawals are balanced with deposits we can create more supportive, responsive environments that prevent burnout, meltdowns or withdrawal, and promote wellbeing and engagement.

Activity

Try drawing out an energy accounting system for a child in your setting: what recharges them (deposits) and what is draining (withdrawals)? Think about if there are enough opportunities for deposits and how these can be implemented across the day.

Top tips for supporting behaviour

- **Change the environment not the child** – This perspective was really emphasised in the fourth parent story in Chapter 2.

We have found educators, and ourselves at times, to be, understandably, focused on changing our daughter's challenging behaviours and increasing her compliance with what we wanted/needed her to do. Three years into our journey, I am now of the view that children this age aren't really able to change themselves or their behaviours. The interventions which reduced her challenging behaviours, and increased her compliance, were working with adults to modify the environment and their expectations of our daughter and supporting her to feel less anxious. In our experience, professionals who focused primarily on stopping her engaging in challenging behaviours caused our daughter to become extremely distressed and more anxious, with an increase in challenging behaviours. Initially we thought that, as experts, they must know what they are doing and that we would be letting our daughter down by not staying the course with these interventions. We now bitterly regret having exposed our daughter to that and fear they will have had a lasting impact on her self-esteem and trust in us.

- **Understand Autism and Autistic thinking** – Trying to get into the shoes of the children you work with will help you in your ability to problem solve what is happening for them. Remember all the theories and concepts we talked about in Chapter 1. Understanding these is key to making sense and problem-solving situations.
- **Be a detective** – Use the iceberg and look for patterns of behaviour and what may be going on under the waterline. Don't miss out on the 'why'. Sometimes when we become familiar with a child and understand lots about Autism, it is quite easy to jump straight to using a strategy without taking time to build up a picture of when behaviours occur. It is always a worthwhile exercise to complete an iceberg and spend time carefully and deliberately thinking about contributory factors.
- **Adapt the environment** – to allow for structure, predictability and consistency. In a lot of Autistic children, this will reduce stress and anxiety.
- **Adapt your communication and interaction style** – individualise your approach to each Autistic child you meet.
- **Don't get focussed on 'stopping a behaviour'** – This is highlighted in the fourth parent story in Chapter 2 when the parent states:

Challenging behaviours can be so shaming for parents. Try not to focus too much on eliminating the behaviour. Instead, be a detective and focus on identifying the 'gaps' and plugging them. In our experience, identifying the subtle 'gaps' got much easier with age. Be realistic about when you will see improvements. Building up skills takes time. There is no magic wand (and people who offer one should be avoided).

- **Tell a child what to do, not what not to do.** This is a powerful and helpful strategy that most people are familiar with when supporting behaviour. If you have children running down a corridor and the adult is shouting 'No running', in essence the children hear 'running' and keep going. Instead, if the adults say 'Walking', they are telling the child clearly and directly what they are expected to be doing.
- **Look after yourself.** This may sound silly, but being bitten, hit or spat at is not fun, even when it is a small person, and it can feel upsetting. Make sure you talk it through with someone, step away from the situation and have a break and a drink. Remember the child is not being unkind to you, they are likely trying to communicate or in a state of stress or overwhelm.

Activity

Instead of thinking 'This is how I will stop *this behaviour*', brainstorm how you will adapt your environment and yourself to minimise the chance of behaviours occurring in the first place.

Chapter 7 summary

- It's important to look beyond behaviour. Punitive approaches do not work and can cause trauma and anxiety in Autistic children.
- Instead, we need to work collaboratively with parents and professionals. Taking time to build a picture and be a detective is a helpful approach.
- The iceberg model is a helpful framework in understanding 'why' a behaviour occurs and providing context.
- A key take away message is to change yourself and the environment, not the child.
- Focus on getting the basics right and ensure that there is good understanding of Autism and Autistic thinking.

Reference

Toudal, M. and Attwood, T. 2024. *Energy Accounting: Stress Management and Mental Health Monitoring for Autism and Related Conditions*. London: Jessica Kingsley Publishers.

8

Next steps

This manual has provided you with an overview of up-to-date theories and perspectives which reflect the neurodiversity paradigm. Hopefully this has enabled you as a reader to dispel any myths around Autism and shift from a view of deficits to that of differences. As educators we need to recognise strengths and differences whilst acknowledging the real barriers that Autistic children and their families face every day.

Hopefully you will take away with you relevant theories and key concepts in particular:

- Double Empathy
- Monotropism
- Autism + Environment = Outcome (Beardon, 2017)
- Understanding the Autistic experience in terms of alexithymia, interoception, masking and holding it all together

The parent stories have highlighted strengths but also very real challenges that come from a lack of support and access to services and funding.

Having read this manual, you can now:

- Apply your theoretical knowledge of Autism to 'get in the shoes' of an Autistic child you work with
- Use the information gathering and iceberg tools to gain insight into individual strengths and differences whilst remembering that each Autistic child is different
- Help Autistic children feel safe and secure by changing the environment
- Recognise that you can 'change yourself and the environment' to support the Autistic children you work with
- Tune into the children that you work with to support connection, shared attention and joy

DOI: 10.4324/9781003627760-8

- Understand that all forms of communication are valid
- Provide opportunities for play and social connection that are affirmative and not seeking to 'change' a child
- Be a detective and try to work out why behaviours occur
- Work collaboratively with families and recognise how important this is

Before coming to an end, it is important to offer some closing reflections to support you in your next steps and moving forward:

- **Seek relevant support** – Find out what local support services families are able to access in your area, the local offer website is usually a good place to start. Be informed of relevant parent support groups and other local agencies that you can link families into. The National Autistic Society runs a range of parent groups including local support groups (area dependent); the details are listed on their website, www.nas.org.
- **Develop your skills** – Access training wherever possible. Autism is an ever-evolving field, and there are always new and different approaches to be aware of. Find out if there are any Autism special schools or resource bases in your area. Do they offer training or opportunities to observe?
- **Make timely referrals** – The provision of health and education services may be reduced depending on your local area. It is important to access SLT, OT or education psychology if required. Ensure that you know the process to refer to local children's services in terms of information needed, referral forms and so on.
- **Document everything** – Documenting meetings, goals and outcomes is important in the process of applying for further support. Without this, it can be difficult to prove what you have put in place and what a child needs.
- **Give things time** – Strategies may not work straightaway. This is an important point and one that I often encounter in settings that have put excellent strategies in place and then feel despondent that they haven't seen immediate results. Allow six weeks before reviewing.
- **Involve parents** – Not only will this allow for consistency in application of strategies, but also parents know their children best. A collaborative approach is always going to be best.
- **Reflect on the skills that you are developing** – You'll find them in yourself through this process and see the difference that you are making.

- **Acknowledge that it can be hard work** – Seek support and discussion from colleagues and relevant professionals to ensure that you are supported in your work. Although it can be hard work, it is extremely rewarding work supporting children to develop their ability to communicate and engage; you can make a real difference in many areas of their lives.
- **Above all be curious** – Keep an open mind, listen to children and their parents and always be curious and ready to challenge your assumptions.

INDEX

Note: Page locators in **bold** refer to tables and page locators in *italic* refer to tables.

For Product Safety Concerns and Information please contact our EU
representative GPSR@taylorandfrancis.com
Taylor & Francis Verlag GmbH, Kaufingerstraße 24, 80331 München, Germany

www.ingramcontent.com/pod-product-compliance
Lightning Source LLC
LaVergne TN
LVHW061945101026
849885LV00034B/357

* 9 7 8 1 0 4 1 0 4 3 0 7 2 *